Tired of Being Tired?

The Doctor Will See You Now

by

James C. Gariti, M.D.

The techniques presented in this book are for informational purposes only. As each individual situation is unique, you should use proper discretion, in consultation with your doctor, before utilizing the information contained in this book. The author expressly disclaims responsibility for any adverse effects that may result from the use or application of the information contained in this book.

Cover by Terri Breese

Table of Contents

Introduction:

Chronic fatigue is a condition affecting millions of Americans. In my office, fatigue is a symptom described by nearly 20% of my patients, and this is typical in many doctors' offices. Why are we so tired? How can we figure out what's going on? How do we start to improve our energy levels and get on with our normal lives? These are difficult questions, and these are the questions I answer in this book.

This book is designed to describe the most common causes of fatigue, and throughout this book, I describe some of the most common medical illnesses that have fatigue as one of their symptoms. I will also list some of the less common medical illnesses that can present with fatigue. I will lead you through the steps you can take toward discovering the cause of your low energy level, and I will describe the medical workup I typically do as I try to figure out why a person is feeling so run down.

Once you know why you're tired, you'll be able to take specific steps toward improving your symptoms and returning to the level of functioning you remember. In this book I'll review the most common treatments for chronic fatigue, and I'll discuss some of the common mistakes people make as they attempt to increase their energy levels. Besides describing the steps you can take on your own to improve identified problems with your energy level, I'll review some of the most common treatments prescribed by physicians for the most common causes of fatigue. I will also look at some of the ways you can increase your energy level in general. The methods I will discuss will include making dietary changes and lifestyle changes as well as utilizing prescription medications, herbs, and vitamins. I will present the best information available regarding these different therapies including their proven and stated advantages and disadvantages.

Introduction

Overall, after having read this book, you will have a better understanding of why you feel like you do. You will be able to look at what treatment options are available and which ones hold the most promise for improving your life. If you feel fine, I encourage you to read this book for information only. But if you are fatigued and you can't do all the things you used to be able to do, I encourage you to follow as many of the following suggestions as closely as possible. And, in the end, I hope that after you correct as many of the fatigue-causing problems in your life as possible, the active, energetic lifestyle you remember from years gone by can become a daily reality for today and into the future.

James C. Gariti, M.D.

Section I: What Causes Fatigue?

What Causes Fatigue?

Chapter 1: Fatigue Defined

Before we can begin any discussion about the common causes of fatigue, we must first be sure that we are talking about the same symptom. Frequently, patients come to me telling me that they are tired, and as we continue our conversation, I discover that what they are experiencing isn't really fatigue but is instead some other symptom that is frequently confused with fatigue. **Fatigue** is defined by Merriam-Webster's dictionary as weariness or exhaustion from labor, exertion, or stress. It relates to a low level of energy. To feel constantly tired, as if you could fall asleep anywhere, anytime would describe fatigue.

It's important to distinguish this low level of energy from some of the nerve and muscle conditions that are often mistaken for fatigue. Muscle weakness, for example, is different from fatigue. **Muscle weakness** is best described as not physically being able to perform routine tasks. With muscle weakness, you have less strength than normal, and after a limited amount of activity, your muscles are unable to perform additional work. For example, normally, when you wake up in the morning, you are able to comb your hair and go up a flight of stairs. Now, after only a few strokes of your hair, you need to rest. Then after climbing only two or three stairs you have no strength left to complete the climb. These would be examples of muscle weakness. The causes, and therefore treatments, for muscle weakness, are vastly different than the causes and treatments for fatigue.

Another symptom that is often confused with fatigue is a lack of concentration. If I ask a patient to spell the word "WORLD" then spell it backwards (DLROW) and if the patient can't complete the task, this would be more typical for a lack of concentration. Another example would be a person who normally begins the day by getting out of bed, drinking a cup of coffee, showering, and dressing. If he now cannot complete the entire

3

sequence of events and instead ends up sitting on the couch watching television with a cup of coffee in hand, that, too, can be a lack of concentration. **Concentration** is the ability to focus on a task until the task is completed. Concentration is important if we are going to finish the tasks of daily living. A lack of concentration is a significant medical finding and can correspond to any number of medical conditions; however, they are very different medical conditions than the ones that cause fatigue.

I frequently see other patients who have difficulty following simple instructions. For example, I might ask a patient to pick up a piece of paper and a pen and then write her name on the piece of paper. In response, the person might take the pen, and after staring at the paper for a period of time she might put the pen back down without having written anything on the paper. This person is also suffering from something other than fatigue. This person was not able to follow these simple instructions, most likely because of a short circuit between the part of the brain that understands speech and the part of the brain that controls her body's movements. The short circuit can occur in the understanding step of completing the task (the brain did not understand all the words that were heard) or in the converting what she heard into actions (the brain tells the hand to move, but the hand doesn't respond). Sometimes a person appears to have difficulty following simple instructions because she lacks the concentration necessary to complete the task. Regardless of the cause, if a person is not able to follow a sequence of simple instructions, that person may have a hard time completing her daily chores. This inability to complete simple tasks is frequently viewed by the person's spouse as laziness (because the chores aren't being done) or fatigue (because the person frequently decides to go to sleep instead of trying to figure out how to complete the tasks). Any of the diseases that cause problems with brain function similar to the problems I just described are significant medical issues that are treated differently than fatigue

There are also many barriers to receiving signals from our surroundings that can often be confused with fatigue. I will never forget visiting my grandparents. As we'd enter the door, my grandmother would yell into the basement "Oh, Jay, the kids are here." Finally, after several more calls and no response, we'd head down the stairs to find my grandfather asleep in front of the television with the volume on the television loud enough for the neighbors to hear it. **Social isolation** due to hearing impairments or vision impairments frequently causes an otherwise normal, healthy, energetic person to spend the majority of his time in a safe, comfortable place (frequently in a chair in front of the television, asleep). He stays in his safe place in order to prevent an awkward or dangerous situation, and because he's essentially bored, he simply falls asleep as a way to pass the time. Hearing and vision impairments can often be overcome. Unfortunately, they are often confused with other medical problems including fatigue.

As you can tell, fatigue isn't always as easy to spot as it might seem. It's frequently discussed, whether over the dinner table or in my office, but it's often confused with things that look like fatigue. The significance, diagnosis, and treatment of many of these other diseases vary, but the importance of recognizing that they are not fatigue is crucial.

For the purposes of this book, I will focus on fatigue. Why don't I have the energy I used to have? Why do I fall asleep as soon as I get home from work? Why do I have such a hard time waking up in the morning? Why would I rather relax on the couch instead of doing the things I used to do? These are fatigue, and throughout the course of this book I will explain the why, what, and   how   of   it.

Fatigue Defined

Chapter 2: Causes of Fatigue—Sleep

As we begin our discussion of fatigue, the first question to ask is, "What do our bodies tell us to do when we're tired?" As we all know, they tell us to go to sleep. Since sleep and fatigue are so closely tied to each other, a person's pattern of sleep is one of the first things I look at when she comes to me with concerns about fatigue. What time does she go to bed? What time does she wake up? Does she sleep all night? If not, why not?

To make sure we're all on the same page, I'm going to provide a description of a normal night's sleep. A normal night's sleep begins with a person feeling tired. This person decides to go to sleep. She then lies down in her bed. Within 15 minutes, she's asleep. Throughout the night, she remains in bed, asleep. In the morning, she awakes, completely rested and full of energy to pursue her day.

In my office, my patients describe tremendous variations on this normal pattern. A common story I might hear sounds something like this: "Doc, I'm tired all the time. When I go to sleep at night I'm tired. When I wake up in the morning I'm tired. Five years ago, I had all the energy I needed, but today, I'm plain worn out." My first question is, "What time do you go to bed?" "Well, Doc, I usually finish watching the news around 11:30, and after I'm done brushing my teeth, I'm in bed by midnight." "What time do you get up in the morning?" "Well, I start work at 6:00, so I'm usually up by 5:00." After just a couple simple questions and answers, the cause of this patient's fatigue is obvious. This poor guy is only getting five hours of sleep each night, and that's a problem.

Our bodies were built with preset schedules for sleeping and waking. These schedules are called **circadian rhythms**. Circadian rhythms are what tell our bodies when it's time to sleep

7

and when it's time to wake up, and these cycles are closely related to the amount of daylight in a given day. Our brains receive this information about daylight, and in response, they release a variety of hormones. These hormones then signal to our consciousness that we should be tired or we should be alert. These internal clocks have a certain amount of time scheduled for sleep, and for most people, that amount of time is roughly eight hours per night. When we were infants and again when we were adolescents, that amount of time increased (to maybe 10 or 12 hours per night). As we enter our later years, that amount of time decreases (to maybe six or seven hours per night). We don't exactly understand what our brains are doing during this preset amount of time or why they require the amount of time they do, but we do know that if we routinely deprive our brains of the amount of sleep they need, they won't be happy. In fact, a lot of research has been done on **sleep deprivation** (not getting enough sleep), and as the degree of sleep deprivation increases the side effects become more and more intense. These side effects can range from fatigue to agitation to anxiety to depression to paranoia to elevated blood pressure to fluid retention.

To understand why the gentleman in our example is tired isn't very difficult. Five hours of sleep each night simply isn't enough to restore his brain to a normal, rested level. For better or worse, our brains are persistent, and they will fight hard to get what they want. Eventually, they will overcome us with their desires. With continued sleep deprivation, we will become so tired that we won't physically be able to stay awake any longer, and at some point, we will be forced to get some sleep. Luckily, our brains have a way of catching up on sleep. This means that, if we deprive our brains of sleep during the week but allow ourselves unlimited amounts of sleep on the weekend, our brains will frequently return to their normal functioning by the end of the weekend. This is a great way to return our brains to their normal rested states. What I see much too often, however, is that, instead of getting caught up on sleep during the weekend, people try to cram all their chores into their precious "free" time. In this situation, people don't get caught up on sleep, and the sleep deprivation worsens. My patients then come to see me, exhausted, and when I suggest they need more sleep, they ask me, "Who has time for sleep?" Trust me—your brain knows if you try to cheat it. Everybody's brain needs the amount of sleep it needs. There's no way around it. Ultimately, giving your brain what it needs (some extra sleep) will go a long way toward eliminating many cases of fatigue.

Another common sleep pattern I see in my office is described by a person who spends a normal amount of time in bed but still doesn't feel rested when she wakes up in the morning. It doesn't always make sense that a person could spend 10 hours each night in bed and still feel tired throughout the following day. This phenomenon is related to what we call the stages of sleep. Doctors have studied the electrical activity of people's brains while they have slept, and they have found several consistently identifiable patterns in the electrical activity. We call these electrical activity patterns **sleep stages**. Throughout the night, our brains travel through different depths of sleep from light sleep to deep sleep as we pass from Stage 1 to Stage 4 sleep. When we first fall asleep, we are still easily arousable (Stage 1), but as time passes, our brains fall deeper into sleep (Stage 2-Stage 4). Then, interestingly, our brains begin to wake again, and just before we are fully awake, our brains experience a phenomenon called **REM (rapid eye movement) sleep**. REM sleep is a sleep stage in which there is an intense amount of brain activity. The brain then cycles itself back down into deep sleep and then back up towards REM sleep. This sequence from Stage 1 to REM and back again is called a **sleep cycle**, and we may experience four or five sleep cycles each night. As the sleep cycles progress throughout the night and toward the morning, there is more and more REM sleep and less and less deep sleep (Stage 4 sleep).

The exact function of each stage of sleep hasn't yet been discovered, but we do know that in childhood we experience more REM and deep sleep than we do as adults. We also know that if a person is sleep-deprived, his brain will experience increased deep sleep at the expense of other forms of sleep when the opportunity is presented. We know that REM sleep is the stage of sleep when we dream, when our minds are most active and our bodies are almost completely inactive. These stages of sleep are likely responsible for restoring and repairing physical and chemical injuries and deficiencies of the brain. We know that, during these different stages of sleep, the brain releases a large variety of different chemicals into the bloodstream, and these chemicals affect the function of the entire body. Again, our understanding of why we travel through these various stages of sleep each night is not complete, and exactly what is happening to our brains and the rest of our bodies during the different stages of sleep isn't fully clear, but it is clear that if we don't complete the number and type and duration of stages of sleep we need, we will feel more and more fatigued as time goes on. So, more than likely, when a person gets out of bed 8 or 10 hours after first lying down and still feels tired, she is experiencing an abnormal pattern of sleep cycles. When we want to quantify and give a name to this concept of how rested a person should feel after spending a certain amount of time in bed, we use a sort of ratio comparing these two numbers. Comparing how rested a person feels to how much time she spent in bed can be described as **sleep efficiency**. A very efficient night's sleep might involve spending six hours in bed and feeling fully rested in the morning, while an inefficient night's sleep might involve feeling exhausted despite having spent 10 hours in bed. Sleep cycles and circadian rhythms are most often hidden contributors to sleep efficiency, and becoming aware of these contributors and understanding how altering them affects both sleep efficiency and daytime energy levels are important steps toward improving fatigue.

Now let's discuss some of the specific causes of abnormal sleep efficiency. A common cause of fatigue that's related to our circadian rhythms and abnormal sleep stages is the difficulty night-shift workers have. These people try to work at night and sleep during the day. Since our circadian rhythms are primarily driven by the day/night cycle, trying to work around what your brain wants you to do can be difficult. When people experience insomnia and fatigue associated with working the night shift, we call this **shift work sleep disorder**. If someone is consistently sleeping when his brain wants him to be awake and staying awake when his brain wants him to sleep, he will quickly notice that falling asleep can be a challenge and staying awake can be nearly impossible. Occasionally, with time and training, the brain can learn to adapt, but it's usually not without difficulty. If you are experiencing shift work sleep disorder, there are things your doctor can do to help you overcome this challenge. There are prescription medications, as well as behavior modifications and vitamin supplements that are commonly used, and I strongly encourage you to discuss the available treatment options with your doctor.

Along these same lines, but even more difficult for our brains to accommodate, is a work or sleep schedule that is constantly changing. Our brains have a difficult time getting used to working the day shift one week, the night shift the next, and third shift the next. We see a similar difficulty in night-shift workers who, throughout the week, sleep during the day but on the weekends try to sleep at night. Whenever the timing of sleep changes, our brains have difficulty adapting to the change, and in return, we may have difficulty maintaining our alertness and functional capacity. Fixing the fatigue associated with changing sleep schedules requires sleeping during the same time of day each day. For those folks who are required to change work shifts periodically, fixing the problem can be very difficult, and often the best option is to discuss with your employer working the same shift on a regular basis. For those folks who sleep during the day throughout the week, continuing the same sleep pattern on weekends can help improve energy levels. If sleeping during the same time each day isn't an option, talking with your doctor and discussing options used to treat shift work sleep disorder will be the next best choice.

Shifting the timing of sleep is the same phenomenon that happens with **jet lag**—our bodies are in one time zone while our brains are in another. As anyone who has experienced jet lag will acknowledge, jet lag produces a sense of fatigue that can interfere with normal functioning when arriving in a new city, and jet lag can drag on for days if not dealt with effectively. Jet lag is a direct result of trying to change our bodies' circadian rhythms, and the most effective treatment for jet lag involves resynchronizing our brains with our bodies. The trick to avoiding the difficulties associated with jet lag is to force ourselves to make this transition as soon as possible. To achieve this, there are two main options: we can either force ourselves to sleep when we are supposed to be sleeping (if it's nighttime in our destination, we need to force ourselves to sleep even if our brains think it's daytime), or we can force ourselves to stay awake when we are supposed to be awake (if it's daytime in our destination, we need to force ourselves to stay awake even if it means staying awake all night and even if it means we end up staying awake for more than 24 hours in a row). For most of us, forcing ourselves to stay awake is easier than forcing ourselves to fall asleep. This means the most effective way for us to overcome and even prevent the potential effects of jet lag is to stay awake until it's bedtime in our new time zone. When facing jet lag, be prepared...you will be tired sometime during the day of your arrival, and you will be tempted to "take a little nap" in an attempt to catch up on sleep. Taking that nap is the biggest potential pitfall you will face because sleeping during daytime hours will only prolong your jet lag. In this situation, it's important to not take a nap, even if you're exhausted. The better choice is to force yourself to stay awake until it's bedtime. This technique will still be effective even if you end up going to bed a little before your normal bedtime (for example, if you usually go to bed at 10pm, you can allow yourself to go to bed at 9pm in your new destination). As I described, you may feel tired the day of your arrival, but when you wake up the next morning, your brain will be synchronized with the day/night schedule of your new location, and this will make the rest of your trip much more enjoyable.

The next sleep-related, fatigue-causing issue we will discuss is insomnia. **Insomnia** is the inability to fall asleep, and while an occasional difficulty falling asleep has happened to all of us, some people deal with it on a daily basis. Insomnia causes a sleep-deprived state, and again, in response, the brain becomes tired which causes our bodies to feel fatigued. Unfortunately for some, as their problems with insomnia increase and their fatigue increases, their preoccupation with their sleep difficulties increases as well. As they think about sleep more and more, almost obsessed with falling asleep, their conscious minds heighten their awareness that they aren't asleep. And as the conscious competes with the unconscious, the insomnia worsens. In time, they are so focused on sleeping that they can't allow their brains to relax enough to fall asleep. It's a terrible cycle causing many people to perform their daily tasks while constantly feeling tired. Finding ways to break this cycle and allowing their brains to fall asleep is critical, and I will discuss some of the methods we use to help insomnia in a later chapter.

Another common cause of sleeping difficulties is the use of stimulant medications before bedtime. I will review the effects of a large variety of medications later in the book, but for now, I will simply introduce the concept of stimulant medications. **Stimulants** are chemicals that cause the brain to be more awake. The most common stimulants we use are caffeine and nicotine. The effects of caffeine can last several hours, so for some, even having a cup of coffee with dinner is enough to keep them tossing and turning all night. **Caffeine** and chemicals similar to caffeine (like **theobromine**, phenylethylamine, **theanin**, and **theophylline**) are found in many of the foods and beverages we commonly eat and drink. Besides watching our evening coffee intake we have to be aware of the quantities of chocolate we eat and how many cups of tea or glasses of soda we drink. Some vitamin supplements, especially those used for weight loss or increased energy or increased attention, contain a variety of different stimulants to achieve these effects which means we have to pay attention to the time of day we take these vitamins and how long the effects last.

For some people, these chemicals have less intense effects which means some people can drink as many cups of coffee as they like right before bed without noticing any impact on their sleep. These people don't need to monitor their stimulant intake. But for those folks struggling with sleeping difficulties, identifying stimulant effects and eliminating the stimulants can often solve their problems.Nicotine is a somewhat unique drug for several reasons. With regards to sleep, it, too, is a potent stimulant and therefore can keep us from falling asleep. Its effects are felt within seconds, and they usually wear off between 30 minutes and 2 hours later. Nicotine dissolves into fat, so smoking on a regular basis creates a stockpile of the drug that is constantly leaking into our bloodstreams. Also, our bodies develop tolerance to nicotine within days of regular use, so it takes more and more nicotine to provide us with the same level of stimulation. If our bodies do not have the amount of nicotine they are used to, they will experience withdrawal. Withdrawal symptoms often include agitation, irritability, insomnia, and headaches. Therefore, a smoker may be experiencing insomnia either due to excessive nicotine intake prior to bedtime or due to withdrawal from nicotine that coincides with bedtime. Ultimately, quitting smoking and stopping the use of all nicotine-containing products are the best steps we can take to prevent or treat a wide range of medical conditions including insomnia and chronic fatigue. For most people who have tried to quit using nicotine, they've discovered that quitting is far from easy. Part of the difficulty is overcoming nicotine withdrawal. The other part of the difficulty is getting out of the "habit" of using tobacco. Smokers tell me they often smoke while in certain situations because they are used to smoking in those situations. For example, many smokers are used to having a cigarette with their first cup of coffee of the day. The routine of smoking while drinking coffee makes it difficult for a smoker to imagine or get used to drinking a cup of coffee without smoking a cigarette. Another situation that makes it difficult for some tobacco users to quit using tobacco is that they have been using nicotine (and other drugs for that matter) to treat undiagnosed medical conditions. For example, **attention deficit hyperactivity disorder (ADHD)** is a

14

medical condition in which a person's brain is too active and the brain bounces from one idea to the next without the person being able to always control when and where the thoughts bounce. As counter intuitive as it might seem, most of the medications used to treat ADHD are stimulants. Stimulants, as it turns out, actually have the opposite effect on the brains of people with ADHD compared to people who do not have ADHD. In people who have ADHD, stimulants cause their brain function to slow down. For people with undiagnosed ADHD who notice they feel more focused and less restless while using tobacco, part of that effect may be due to the fact that nicotine is acting as a stimulant treatment. For these people, replacing nicotine with a longer-acting, most likely prescription, stimulant may ultimately lead to better focus and possibly better sleep. For most tobacco users, either because of long-term nicotine use or because of other underlying medical conditions, quitting using nicotine is very difficult. Most tobacco users make multiple attempts to quit before they finally succeed. Understanding how difficult it is for most people to quit using tobacco and understanding that there are other circumstances that can make quitting even more difficult, it makes sense that a person who has tried to quit but who has not yet been successful should seek any and all forms of assistance available, including discussing the options for quitting with his doctor, as well as looking for other counseling and support groups. Continuing to try to quit and trying different techniques to help with quitting are the keys to eventual success.

Alcohol is another chemical that can have profound effects on both sleep and fatigue. I frequently see patients who tell me that they have a beer or two before bed to help them relax and fall asleep. Alcohol is a **depressant** meaning it slows down brain function. Alcohol reduces mental function, relaxes us, and will help us fall asleep. Unfortunately, it also prevents the brain from going through its normal sleep cycles. After a couple drinks, the brain experiences less deep sleep and more frequent nocturnal awakenings, and, as described above, the brain doesn't like being cut short on deep sleep. With time and the repeated use of alcohol as a sleep aid, fatigue will increase and sleeping difficulties will worsen. Alcohol also has many of the tolerance and withdrawal issues described above with nicotine. This translates into the fact that a person who routinely uses a couple beers to help himself fall asleep may need more and more alcohol over time to obtain the same effect. Additionally, it's not uncommon to have a very difficult time sleeping without alcohol, and in the absence of alcohol, withdrawal symptoms, including restlessness and anxiety, may occur, further impairing his ability to sleep. Eventually, he may become completely dependent on alcohol to get any amount of sleep, and he will take what sleep he can get even if that sleep is non-refreshing. It's not a healthy pattern to get into, and it's not an easy one to get out of. This means that it's better to not start using alcohol to help with sleep, and if you're already doing this, it's better to quit, deal with the withdrawal (which will be short-lived), and move toward better, more restful sleep. As with nicotine, quitting using alcohol can be difficult. Withdrawal can be intense, and some people are using alcohol to treat undiagnosed medical conditions (again, like ADHD and depression). These factors can make it difficult to quit drinking, and it makes sense to use all the help available, including your doctor, counselors, and support groups to increase your chances of success.

Another common cause of sleep difficulties is medication use. Medications, both over-the-counter and prescription, both natural and synthetic, commonly cause complicated sleep patterns. Many of the medications we frequently use, especially those for blood pressure, mood changes, allergies, seizures, and Parkinson's disease, can increase daytime sleepiness (and therefore reduce nighttime sleepiness). Many medications and herbal supplements interfere with the normal stages of sleep. While every medication, vitamin, and herb is being taken with the intention of helping us in some way, they all have associated side effects. To make the situation more complicated, we often end up taking another medication to help reduce these side effects. The more medications we add on top of each other, the more complex the chemistry becomes and the more likely we are to have even more side effects. In order to decide whether or not to continue using all these medications, you need to weigh the benefits you are getting against the side effects you are experiencing. This is one of those situations in which less is more, and the fewer medications (again, including prescriptions, over-the-counter, herbal supplements, and vitamins) we take, the better off we usually are. As we age there is an increased likelihood of being on at least one medication that will adversely affect sleep. These medications are often necessary for our overall health, but they can leave us fatigued.   Weighing the benefits and side effects can be difficult, and finding a suitable alternative isn't always easy. This is the point where reviewing the medications with your doctor or your pharmacist can be very helpful.

Besides understanding that a variety of different chemicals can stimulate the brain and make it more difficult for us to fall asleep, we must also recognize that some of the activities that we perform can do the same thing. All of us have had the experience of trying to fall asleep after having watched a scary movie...our hearts are pounding, and every creak of a floor board conjures up the image of an intruder just on the other side of the bedroom door. Our minds become so focused on that door and the imaginary intruder on the other side that falling asleep becomes virtually impossible. This excited state is caused by our bodies' release of **adrenaline** (also known as epinephrine), and adrenaline is a stimulant. The effects of adrenaline are just like those of any other stimulant, and they include increased mental alertness which makes it much more difficult to sleep. Adrenaline is a hormone our bodies produce as part of a protective instinct called the **fight or flight response**. The fight or flight response is one mechanism our brains and bodies use to deal with life-threatening situations in which immediate action is required to survive. It's a reflex, and it happens immediately and automatically and is, for the most part, out of the control of our conscious minds. When we are faced with a life-threatening situation, we are hardwired to either fight against the threat or run away from it (therefore the term "fight or flight"). This protective response originally allowed us to act quickly when

17

a saber tooth tiger jumped out from behind a rock and threatened to eat us. Whenever we hear about someone demonstrating "superhuman" strength in an emergency situation, this is the mechanism responsible. Activities that cause adrenaline release typically delay our transition into sleep. These activities can range from exercise to watching TV to playing games to having intense conversations to reading interesting books, so avoiding stimulation before bedtime can be a key way of improving sleep efficiency. Exercise is somewhat unique because it has the potential to both stimulate and relax us. Exercise causes our bodies to release a variety of different hormones into our bloodstreams including adrenaline, but among the other chemicals potentially released by the brain with exercise are **endorphins** which make us relax and feel happy. Because these chemicals can be released in different amounts with different exercises, exercise can cause some people to stay awake at night and can help others fall asleep more easily. As a general rule, if you are having difficulty falling asleep at night, avoid exciting activities in the evening including exercise. Instead, get into the habit of spending extra time relaxing immediately before bedtime. Try meditating or taking a hot shower or bath. Ten minutes of relaxation just before trying to fall asleep can stimulate endorphin release by the brain, can give your mind time to process any lingering thoughts from the day and can send a signal to your brain that it's time to shut down and prepare for sleep. Getting into this habit can be remarkably effective at improving sleep quality and can be crucial for anyone struggling to get a good night's rest.

As a rule, our brains like routines. They get used to performing certain activities in certain ways at certain times. These routines include falling asleep. We'll talk more about this topic later in the book, but for now, I'll introduce the concept that not sleeping at night can be caused by getting your brain used to sleeping at other times of the day. Napping, although it may feel good at the time, actually disrupts our normal sleep cycles. It sends incorrect signals about timing and duration of sleep to our brains, and our brains, in response, often keep us awake when we should be asleep. People with insomnia will frequently attempt to catch up on sleep by napping during the day, and people who come home from work exhausted will commonly take a quick nap before or after dinner. Unfortunately, this practice of sleeping during "non-sleep" hours reinforces the incorrect sleep habits within our brains and only worsens nighttime sleep difficulties. The primary way we correct this problem is to avoid sleeping during "non-sleeping" hours.

Other habits that adversely affect proper sleep patterns involve using a bed for something it wasn't intended for. Many of us like to lie in bed and read a good book or finish up a little work before we go to sleep. Many people will watch the evening news or a late-night entertainment program while lying in bed. Again, our brains want to perform the same activities in the same places at the same times, so if a person is having a hard time falling asleep, some of that problem can be caused by the person's brain not knowing what to expect when it gets into bed. If we want to train our brains to slow down and fall asleep when we go to bed, the bed should be primarily for sleep. When we use it for other activities, we send incorrect signals to our brains, and our brains, in return, send incorrect signals back to our bodies worsening insomnia.

For many people, the primary issue they deal with is falling asleep, but for others, the problem is staying asleep. Some people are able to fall asleep initially, but for one reason or another they wake up repeatedly throughout the night. Interestingly, these people may not wake to the point of full consciousness each time, so they may not fully realize that they're not sleeping well. They'll only know that they were in bed the whole night and still feel tired in the morning. For many people, waking is caused by too much noise or light in the bedroom (whether it's a bed partner snoring or traffic on a road outside the home or a clock ticking in the background). A simple treatment for trying to sleep in a room with too much noise or light is to wear earplugs and a sleep mask while sleeping. Earplugs and sleep masks have provided numerous patients with significantly improved nights' sleep with no side effects.

For others, interrupted sleep is due to more complex medical conditions. One common medical condition that affects sleep is **obstructive sleep apnea (OSA).** OSA is a condition in which the muscles in the back of the throat relax so much when a person falls asleep that the skin in the back of the throat blocks air from flowing into the lungs. This most commonly happens in people who have extra skin in the backs of their throats. Commonly, people with obstructive sleep apnea are obese, have large tongues, have small jaws, and may have large tonsils. One of the best ways to first identify a person with obstructive sleep apnea is to talk to his bed partner. Loud snoring and episodes of completely stopped breathing or choking are typical. A person with obstructive sleep apnea is fatigued because of the disrupted sleep cycles, and the bed partner is also usually fatigued because she wakes up with fear every time the other person stops breathing. We'll talk a lot more about different treatment options for interrupted sleep later in the book, but for now, we'll just say that this repetitive waking at night leaves a person exhausted the next day, even if the total number of hours spent in bed should have been adequate.

Another common medical condition that can cause a poor sleep pattern and chronic fatigue is inadequate lung function. Our brains have very sensitive oxygen and carbon dioxide sensors. (Carbon DIoxide is not to be confused with carbon MONoxide. **Carbon dioxide** is a normal waste product our bodies produce as we convert food into energy. **Carbon monoxide** is a waste product generated when something like natural gas or wood is burned.) In the human body, when the oxygen level is low or the carbon dioxide level is high in the blood, our brains normally stimulate us to breathe more rapidly or more deeply. Lung tissue is built just like a sponge with little air spaces spread throughout the more solid portions. As blood flows through the solid portions of the lung, oxygen soaks into the blood from the air spaces and carbon dioxide floats out of the blood into the air spaces. This means that breathing allows oxygen to enter the blood and carbon dioxide to leave the blood. If the air spaces of the lungs get filled up with fluid or if the solid portions of the lungs get injured, the movement of oxygen and carbon dioxide into and out of the lungs doesn't happen correctly leading to a variety of major health problems. Along these lines, there are several diseases that can cause either carbon dioxide to be high or oxygen to be low, and we will review some of these now.

One of the most common causes of inadequate breathing is emphysema. **Emphysema**, also referred to as **chronic bronchitis** or **chronic obstructive pulmonary disease (COPD)**, is a disease in which the solid portions of the lung tissue are progressively destroyed (typically by cigarette smoking) leaving less and less area for the blood to flow through the lungs. Once enough lung tissue has been destroyed, the lungs aren't able to bring in enough oxygen or let out enough carbon dioxide. Low oxygen levels or high carbon dioxide levels can cause fatigue by themselves. To compound the problem, when we sleep, we tend to not breathe as deeply or as frequently as we do when we are awake. Therefore, if a person is having difficulties bringing in enough oxygen to begin with because he has emphysema, and he then reduces his breathing effort when he sleeps, he almost assuredly will not bring in adequate oxygen. When there is inadequate oxygen in his blood, his brain will stimulate him to wake up and take a deep breath. He will then fall asleep again. The repeated awakening throughout the night in order to take deep breaths prevents his brain from experiencing its necessary sleep cycles and can lead to increased fatigue.

A similar phenomenon occurs in the disease called **congestive heart failure (CHF)**. In this disease, the heart cannot pump enough blood forward through the body, so the blood backs up. When the blood backs up enough, fluid begins to leak into the air spaces of the lungs. This fluid in the lungs can block oxygen from entering and carbon dioxide from exiting the blood. As with people with emphysema, people with congestive heart failure can have low oxygen levels and can feel fatigued all the time, and this low oxygen state can be worse while asleep.

Another very common sleep disorder that can lead to chronic fatigue is waking at night to go to the bathroom. One reason we need to go to the bathroom more at night is because the kidneys get more blood flow and create more urine when we lay down. This means our bladders fill at a faster rate while we are sleeping which means they may need to be emptied more often. Increased fluid intake during the day can lead to increased urine output at night. Hydration is a key to staying healthy, so I almost never recommend decreasing fluid intake; however, monitoring fluid intake (as we'll describe later in this book) may give you some insight into your daytime drinking habits and how they correlate with your nocturnal urinary habits.

Besides having to deal with more urine being produced at night, as men age, their prostates enlarge which can also impact bladder filling and emptying. The **prostate** is a gland that wraps around the bottom of the bladder (called the **bladder neck**). In some men, as the prostate enlarges, it squeezes the bladder neck and blocks the urine from coming out. This enlargement is usually caused by a disease known as **benign prostatic hypertrophy (BPH)**. BPH, as the name implies, is not a cancerous growth but is rather a benign growth of a portion of the prostate. In men with BPH, the bladder is capable of squeezing hard enough to get some of the urine out, but it cannot get it all out. This means that these men never fully empty their bladders. Since the bladder never fully empties, it doesn't take as much urine to fill it up again. This translates into less and less time between having to go to the bathroom which may lead to men waking several times each night. Treating this blockage with either medications or surgery can allow the bladder to empty more completely thereby reducing the number of times a man might need to go to the bathroom during the night. If you're a man and are waking frequently at night to go to the bathroom, discussing your symptoms and the available treatment options for BPH with your doctor is a good place to start looking for a solution to your problem.

Women can have problems with waking frequently at night to urinate as well. In women, their bladders can change positions inside their bodies. The reason for this is that the muscles in the pelvis help support the bladder, and if these muscles weaken, the bladder may have less support and may begin to move. Weakening of these muscles typically occurs after delivering babies. Estrogen levels also have an effect on the strength of these muscles, and as women go through menopause, there is less estrogen to help keep these muscles strong. A change in bladder position can lead to increased urination at night for women in two ways. The first involves a bladder that empties too easily (called **stress urinary incontinence**). As the bladder shifts, it can move into a position that partially opens the bladder neck and causes the valve that closes the bladder (called the **urinary or bladder sphincter**) to open too easily. Once the bladder fills part way, the sphincter may not be able to hold the urine in. If this happens, the urine can start to leak out of the bladder without the woman expecting it. Anticipating this possibility and wanting to avoid unexpected urine leakage, the woman may decide to go to the bathroom more frequently in order to prevent it. The second occurs when there is a kink in the bladder neck. This blockage in a woman's bladder can act just like an enlarged prostate in a man's bladder. If there's a kink in the bladder neck, the bladder never fully empties, so it remains partially filled, even immediately after urination. If the bladder is continually partially filled, there is less room for new urine to enter the bladder, and it takes less time to fill the bladder which means less time between trips to the bathroom. The end result is that these changes in a woman's urinary habits can cause significant interference with her sleep schedule which can lead to fatigue. If a woman is waking frequently at night to go to the bathroom, there's a variety of different options available to improve bladder position and function, from medications to exercises to surgical and non-surgical procedures. Discussing these options with your doctor will give you an idea of the range of treatments for your particular problem, and taking this step may lead you down the path toward improving your fatigue.

There's another form of urinary incontinence that can affect sleep. In a normally-functioning urinary bladder, as urine enters the bladder, the muscles in the wall of the bladder relax and allow more urine to continue to enter until the bladder is full. When the bladder is full, it sends a signal to the brain letting the brain know that the bladder needs to be emptied. When someone decides to empty her bladder, her brain "tells" her sphincter muscle to relax, and her brain "tells" the bladder muscles to squeeze. Sphincter relaxation combined with bladder muscle contraction leads to urine flowing from the bladder. Each of the steps in this sequence must occur correctly in order for us to have control over our urination. For some people, their bladder muscles have a hard time relaxing, and as soon as the muscles of the bladder start to stretch, they can spasm. We call this condition **overactive bladder**, and it can affect both men and women. What happens to the bladder muscles in a person with an overactive bladder is similar to what happens to the thigh muscles when a doctor taps the knee with that little rubber hammer. The doctor taps the knee, and the foot kicks forward. Just like the tapping of the knee causes an unconscious, uncontrollable movement of the foot, the stretching of the bladder can cause an unconscious, uncontrollable spasm of the bladder in people with overactive bladders. If the spasm is powerful enough, some urine may leak. We call this condition **urge urinary incontinence**. Just like with other urinary difficulties, urge urinary incontinence can directly wake men and women if the bladder spasms are strong enough, and it can indirectly cause men and women to wake as they make an effort to prevent nocturnal urinary leakage. There are several medications that can be prescribed by your doctor that are effective for the treatment of urge urinary incontinence. Depending on the symptoms you are experiencing, your doctor may simply start you on medications, or he may refer you to a **urologist** (a doctor who specializes in the function of the bladder, kidneys, and the rest of the urinary system) for additional diagnostic testing and treatment. If you are experiencing urinary difficulties that are affecting your sleep, the best place to start is with a visit to your doctor to discuss your symptoms and to map out the best treatment strategy for you.

One of the more common causes of abnormal nocturnal urinary habits is a change in hormone levels in women going through menopause. This is one link between inadequate sleep and menopause. Another is hot flashes. Oftentimes, hot flashes are particularly noticeable at night, during sleep. These hot flashes, and the associated night sweats, can have profound effects on the sleep patterns of menopausal women, and seeking ways to improve or eliminate these symptoms is a common goal for most of these women. The symptoms of menopause are caused by inconsistent levels of estrogen being produced by the ovaries. Menopausal ovaries may release a normal amount of estrogen for a period of time, and then, suddenly and unpredictably, they may stop producing estrogen all together. Without estrogen, the woman's body will begin to go through withdrawal, and it's this withdrawal that causes the symptoms of menopause. The most effective treatment for withdrawal from any medication is to give the body the medication it craves. This means the most effective treatment for menopause is to give the body estrogen. Extensive research has been performed on estrogen replacement therapy (or **hormone replacement therapy** (**HRT**)), and this research has created controversy among doctors. Thoughts and opinions about HRT in general have changed greatly over the past several years, and the safety and efficacy of specific hormones have become the topics of intense debate.

Some doctors feel that **bio-identical hormones** (hormones that are commercially produced and are designed to "look" just like the hormones that are produced by a woman's ovaries) are the best options. The preference for bio-identical hormones is usually based on the premise that hormones that "look" like human hormones should work better at controlling menopausal symptoms and should be safer for women to take. Unfortunately, at this point in time, this is just a theory, and we are still waiting for good scientific proof. Another unique aspect of bio-identical hormones is that they are typically produced and sold by small **compounding pharmacies** (pharmacies that essentially make their own medications). These pharmacies have the flexibility to manufacture a specific mixture of hormones for an individual patient, and it's the customized formulation that's attractive for many patients and doctors. It's this same variability that's a source of concern for other doctors as well as for the Food and Drug Administration (FDA). (You can investigate the FDA's opinions in more detail by going to www.fda.gov and searching for "bio-identical hormones.") In general, the limitations of smaller pharmacies are that they do not have the same production and testing equipment used by larger pharmaceutical manufacturers, and they do not follow the same standardized processes. This lack of standardization can mean the quality, consistency, and safety of the medications produced and sold by compounding pharmacies may not be at the same level as those produced by the large pharmaceutical manufacturers. Also, compounding pharmacies and the medications they sell are not monitored or regulated by the FDA. The primary function of the FDA is to ensure that medications sold in the United States are safe and effective, but for whatever reason, the FDA does not monitor medications produced by compounding pharmacies. For most medications, the FDA reviews mountains of information about its safety and efficacy before it can be sold in the United States. This is not the case with medications produced by compounding pharmacies. Most medications have been tested on tens or hundreds of thousands of people over many years using very strict research protocols before they are presented to the FDA for approval. Again, this is not the case with medications produced by compounding pharmacies. Once a medication is approved, the FDA performs ongoing monitoring of commercial pharmaceutical manufacturers to ensure the medications being produced continue to be safe and effective over time. Once again, this is not the case with medications produced by compounding pharmacies. Even with FDA review and oversight, unexpected side effects and complications can arise.

Without FDA monitoring, the safety and efficacy of a medication are even less sure. Many doctors prefer to know what to expect when they prescribe a medication to a patient, so the level of unpredictability associated with compounded medications can be unsettling for them.

If compounded, bio-identical hormones are on one side of the HRT discussion, the pharmaceutical versions of hormones are on the other. The large pharmaceutical manufacturers use hormones that "look" different than human hormones. These estrogens have been used to treat menopausal symptoms for more than 70 years, and billions of women have taken these preparations over that period of time. It's this extensive experience that has given many doctors a level of comfort with prescribing these hormones for their patients. These estrogens are usually taken from plants or animals and made into medications for humans, and while the effects of these substances appear to be similar to those of human hormones, questions have been raised about potential hazards associated with using non-human hormones in the human body. At this time, the question of elevated risk remains, but just the possibility of additional adverse outcomes has led many doctors away from using these products. There are many doctors on each side of this issue, and the information you receive about HRT will depend on your doctor's opinion, as well as your particular medical situation. Unfortunately, we don't know for certain what the "truth" is regarding the best way to use HRT, so deciding whether or not to use it, as well as what type to use, is based on imperfect information. In situations like this, the best strategy is to sit down with your doctor and discuss the risks and benefits of all the options and then choose the one that's most comfortable for you. Also, don't hesitate to bring the topic up for discussion periodically so you can stay up-to-date on current information. This will help to ensure you remain comfortable with your selection over time.

For those folks for whom HRT isn't the answer, there are some alternatives. In general, these alternatives are not as effective as replacing the missing estrogen, but for some women, the symptoms of menopause can be adequately controlled with non-hormonal therapies. Among these options, some antidepressants (Effexor® in particular) have been shown to be effective treatments for hot flashes and night sweats, not to mention many of the other symptoms of menopause. Also, various herbal supplements (especially black cohosh, red clover, dong quai, soy products, ginseng, and ginkgo biloba) have been promoted as providing relief for menopausal symptoms. Some of these herbal products are thought to increase a woman's own estrogen production, and some may have antidepressant effects. As is the case with most herbal supplements, the research surrounding the risks and benefits of using these products is limited. This means we do not know, with any degree of certainty, that they provide true relief for menopausal symptoms, and we do not know if they are safe to be taken by women who are going through menopause. These medications may be safe or they may not. These medications may relieve menopausal symptoms, or they may just be placebos. (A **placebo** is a simulated treatment for a medical condition. The treatment has no true effect on the medical condition, but it's designed to make the person think she is receiving an effective treatment. The person may experience a perceived or real improvement in the symptoms. Placebos are commonly used in research studies in order to test which effects and side effects are being caused by a medication and which are being caused by a person's mind.) Whether these herbal supplements are safe and whether they're more effective than placebos, we simply don't know. What we do know is that many women use herbal supplements to control their menopausal symptoms, so they deserve consideration when looking for a non-hormonal treatment for hot flashes. Whether it's HRT or non-hormonal alternatives, no one treatment option is perfect for everyone, so discussing the advantages and disadvantages of each with your doctor is the best way to proceed through the maze that leads to the best solution for your menopausal symptoms.

Besides urinary symptoms and hormonal changes waking people at night, there are several other diseases that adversely affect sleep patterns. Many people suffer from **restless leg syndrome (RLS)**—a disease characterized by any of a number of sensations including burning, itching, tingling, crawling, or tightening in the legs that make the person feel as if they have to move the legs in order to relieve the symptoms. The causes of RLS are not well understood, and the treatments for RLS vary greatly. Some cases of RLS are caused by abnormal brain or nerve activity. Some are caused by abnormal skin function. Some are caused by abnormal muscle function. Some are likely caused by vitamin or mineral deficiencies. And some are caused by varicose and spider veins. At some point in the future, we will develop tests to diagnose the specific cause of each person's RLS symptoms, and we will be able to treat the specific cause appropriately. For now, if you find that you awake at night with uncomfortable feelings in your legs and you need to walk for a while in order for the sensations to go away, you likely have RLS. For my patients with RLS, I prefer to look for the simple solutions first, so I typically start out with compression stockings. Wearing compression stockings during the day improves vein function. If wearing the compression stockings during the day improves your RLS symptoms at night, your RLS is likely being caused by abnormal veins. RLS caused by vein problems should respond almost immediately once you start using the compression stockings. In this case, you can either continue to use the compression stockings indefinitely, or you can have your varicose and spider veins treated. If the compression stockings don't help, I usually recommend my patients start taking a multivitamin if they aren't already. If the RLS is being caused by a vitamin deficiency, the RLS symptoms should improve within a month of taking a daily multivitamin. If there is no improvement with regular use of a multivitamin, the final simple treatment for RLS is to keep the skin moist in order to reduce irritation in the skin. Skin moisturizing is best achieved by applying a thick cream to the skin immediately after a bath or shower and again one or two more times during the day. Some people's skin can be irritated by dyes or perfumes that are added to many skin creams, so using a dye-free, perfume-free cream is the best choice. If your case of RLS is being caused by skin irritation, it should improve within a month of regular moisturizing cream application. If it doesn't improve, you need to consider other treatment options, and this will require a visit to your doctor. At this point, I typically move on to a trial of one of the several medications currently used to treat the nerve and other causes of RLS. Unfortunately, finding the right medication can take some experimentation, and it can take time. This means that patience and persistence are key in working through the process of finding a successful treatment for RLS symptoms. Since RLS has such a wide variety of causes and treatments, finding the right treatment for your cause will take time, but once an effective treatment is identified, it will be worth the effort because elimination of RLS symptoms typically translates into improved sleep efficiency and improved daytime energy levels.

Another common nocturnal event that prevents people from getting a good night's sleep is leg cramps. **Leg cramps** are frequently experienced during sleep and most commonly affect the calf muscles (although the feet and thighs can cramp as well). Leg cramps at night are most often caused by varicose and spider veins, and a trial of compression stockings during the day along with leg muscle stretching before bed are very likely to reduce or eliminate the cramping at night. Besides vein problems, leg cramps can occur for a variety of other reasons as well, although in these cases, symptoms increase with activity rather than with rest. Active muscles need increased blood flow. If there's an inadequate amount of blood flowing into the muscles during these times, the muscles will start to cramp. One of the most common causes of inadequate blood flow is dehydration. We'll discuss dehydration in more detail later, but for now, it's important to understand that **dehydration** is associated with decreased amounts of blood in our circulation. With a decreased amount of blood circulating, there's less blood available to carry oxygen, and with less oxygen available for active muscles, their typical response is to cramp. Unfortunately, many of us don't drink enough fluids on a daily basis, and we live with a baseline state of mild dehydration. We can tolerate this mild form of dehydration during normal daily activities, but with increased activity this mild dehydration can worsen which can lead to leg cramps. Again, we'll discuss the best ways to approach dehydration in a later chapter, but for now, the main focus for treating or, better yet, preventing dehydration is to increase our fluid intake. If increased fluid intake resolves your leg cramps, your leg cramps were most likely caused by dehydration, and maintaining your increased fluid intake is the best way to prevent your leg cramps in the future. We see similar episodes of leg cramps (mostly with activity and occasionally at rest) with certain electrolyte deficiencies (different salts like sodium, potassium, calcium, magnesium, and chloride are referred to as **electrolytes**). Increasing our electrolyte intake (either through sports drinks or vitamin supplements) can improve leg cramps caused by electrolyte deficiencies, but these deficiencies are less common. Because electrolyte deficiencies are uncommon, be aware that, if increasing your electrolyte intake improves your leg cramps, it may be a sign that some other disease process is at work, and it will be important to work with your doctor to find the cause. Severe, undiagnosed cases of electrolyte deficiencies can be life threatening, and identifying them and treating them appropriately can prevent long-term complications. Unfortunately, leg cramps are very common, and they can prevent us from experiencing a good-night's sleep. A trial of compression stockings during the day, increased water intake throughout the day, and leg stretches before bed can reduce or eliminate most nocturnal leg cramps. If these basic techniques don't reduce the number or frequency of leg cramps, try increasing your electrolyte intake, and consider seeing your doctor for lab testing and to discuss other possible causes of your symptoms.

The final area I want to discuss in this chapter is chronic pain. Arthritis is associated with an ache in our joints that causes us to move frequently during the night in order to relieve the pain. Chronic back pain can cause us to suffer and remain awake throughout the night, regardless of the position we put our bodies in. In some circumstances, pain in a certain body part makes it impossible to comfortably lie in our favorite sleeping positions. There are numerous techniques available to reduce pain. Besides over-the-counter pain medications, ice or heat application can often improve localized pain. Stretching and low-impact exercise can improve muscle strength and flexibility and reduce joint pain. Meditation and relaxation techniques have been used for centuries to help relieve pain. Massage therapists, chiropractors, and acupuncturists provide reliable pain relief for many patients. Controlling pain can be very important, not only to improving sleep, but also to improving routine daily functioning. If chronic pain is adversely affecting your life and some of the ideas listed above have not provided adequate relief, consider discussing other pain relieving options with your doctor.

Sleep problems are by far the most common causes of fatigue, and as you can see, there are numerous conditions that can lead to inadequate sleep. Becoming familiar with the normal characteristics of sleep, understanding the situations that adversely affect sleep, and working on improving sleep quality are important steps we can all take toward increased energy levels. As we proceed through this book, we'll discuss many more steps we can take to improve our daytime energy levels, but fixing problems with sleep should always remain at the top of our lists.

Chapter 3: Causes of Fatigue— Circulation

Up to this point, we have focused on sleep issues as the primary causes of fatigue because they are the most common causes. However, there are many other reasons why fatigue can begin to dominate a person's life. In the next few chapters, I will explore some of these. Many of the problems discussed in the previous chapter are things you can evaluate and try to correct at home, by yourself. The conditions I will discuss in the following chapters, however, usually require a visit to your doctor and some degree of testing in order to diagnose and treat them. Many of the diseases mentioned in these chapters are complex. They are often difficult to diagnose, and, in some cases, they are challenging to treat effectively. I consider these chapters an advanced course in fatigue. After having read them, you will have a fairly thorough understanding of many of the potential causes of fatigue. You will have been introduced to many of the diseases I consider when I see a patient with fatigue in my office, and this should help you better understand some of the thoughts your doctor is having as he works through the process of diagnosing the cause of your fatigue.

To begin our exploration of non-sleep-related causes of fatigue, we will look at our heart's role in maintaining energy levels. As we begin our discussion of the heart's function within the body and how the heart can make us feel fatigued, I think it's important to review some of the main functions of the heart. To begin with, the heart is relatively easy to understand if we think of it as a pump. It takes blood from one part of the body and pumps it to other parts of the body. By pumping blood around the body, it passes oxygen and nutrients to the various parts of the body which require the oxygen and nutrients for energy. After the energy is used, there are waste products that are put back into the blood. The heart continues to pump the blood (with the waste products) to the parts of the body that clean the blood and get rid of the waste products.

A typical circuit of blood flow might start off in the heart and go to the lungs. While the blood is in the lungs it picks up oxygen. The blood then returns from the lungs back to the heart where it is passed on to the stomach and the rest of the intestines. Here, it picks up the food and other nutrients we have eaten. Now that the blood has oxygen, food, and all the other nutrients, it flows to the muscles, fat, skin, brain, and other organs. These body parts use the oxygen, food, and nutrients as energy and perform whatever functions they are supposed to perform. After using the energy, there are waste products produced. These waste products are put back into the blood, and the blood, with all the waste products, then flows to the kidneys and liver where many of the waste products are cleaned out of the blood. The blood then flows back to the heart. The heart now pumps the blood to the lungs again where the final waste product (carbon dioxide) is removed. Oxygen is replaced at the same time, and the cycle starts over again.

You might wonder how the heart can keep track of which blood is clean and full of energy and which blood is dirty and needs to be cleaned. The answer is that these tasks happen simultaneously to all the blood flowing around the entire body. The lungs, for example, receive the blood from the heart, and while in the lungs, the blood releases its waste products into the air spaces in the lungs and at the same time picks up fresh oxygen from the same air spaces in the lungs. As the blood passes through the muscles, oxygen and nutrients are delivered to the muscle cells at the same time that waste products are collected from the muscle cells. It's absolutely amazing that our bodies manage to perform these functions continually every second of every hour of every day of our lives. As long as each part of the body does its job correctly, we feel fine; however, if one part begins to have trouble, the rest of the body can feel the effects. If, for example, the heart isn't able to pump the blood around the body as well as it needs to, we experience a variety of symptoms. Similarly, if the lungs, the kidneys, or the liver don't remove the waste products well enough, we will have symptoms.

We'll now take a look at some of the abnormal functioning of different body parts that can lead to fatigue, and we'll begin by discussing abnormal functioning of the heart and in particular, abnormalities of the pumping function of the heart. The heart is like a balloon. It has an outer wall with a space in the middle. Its wall is made of muscle, and the space in the middle is filled with blood. The muscular wall of the heart is what squeezes the blood out of the space in the middle. The heart normally pumps in two stages. The first stage is a time of relaxation in which the muscle of the heart relaxes and the space inside the heart fills with blood. The second stage is the time when the heart muscle contracts and squeezes the blood out of the space. When the heart has problems with either the filling or the squeezing stage, this is called **congestive heart failure (CHF)**. Ultimately, whether the blood doesn't come in normally or doesn't go out normally, it backs up, waiting to get through the heart. As the blood backs up, there's increased pressure on the tubes that hold the blood (called the **blood vessels**), and if the pressure gets to be high enough, some of the water that's normally in the blood vessels can leak out. The water can leak out of any of the blood vessels in any of the areas of the body, but one of the most common places this occurs is into the air spaces of the lungs. If enough of the water leaks into the air spaces in the lungs, the water can take up some of the space in the lungs that is normally filled with air thereby reducing the amount of air we are able to breathe in and out of the lungs. If we can't breathe enough air in or out of the lungs, we can't get enough oxygen into the blood or enough carbon dioxide out of the blood. Either low oxygen or high carbon dioxide levels can cause a person's brain to feel fatigued. Also, even if the air spaces in the lungs are completely open, if the heart isn't pumping effectively, there may not be enough blood circulating through the lungs to bring adequate oxygen to or take adequate carbon dioxide from the different body parts and allow those body parts to work normally.

Inadequate blood flow into and out of different body parts can cause a person to feel extremely fatigued, especially when he tries to engage in any amount of activity. Ultimately, whether the heart isn't relaxing enough or contracting enough, the end result and the symptoms are very similar; however, understanding the specific cause of a person's congestive heart failure can help us decide which treatments are most likely to provide the most benefits. I will explain these two types of congestive heart failure and their treatments in more detail next.

When a normal heart muscle relaxes, the space inside the heart can fill with about four ounces of blood. If the walls of the heart are thick or not as stretchy as they should be, the space in the middle can't fill with as much blood, but the amount of blood returning from the body stays the same. Just like trying to force water through a hose with a kink in it, trying to force blood into a heart that is already full creates increased pressure in the blood vessels leading into the heart (we call the blood vessels leading into the heart **veins**). When there's increased pressure in the veins, fluid can leak out of the veins, and it can start to build up in the lungs. As we discussed earlier, this, along with the reduced blood flowing through the heart to the rest of the body, causes fatigue. When the heart muscle cannot relax enough to allow a normal amount of blood to enter it, this leads to a type of congestive heart failure that we call **diastolic dysfunction** (**diastole** (pronounced dī-ás-stō-lē) is the portion of the heart beat when the heart muscle is relaxing). The treatment of diastolic dysfunction is focused on relaxing the heart muscle, and we typically use blood pressure medications to achieve this. Getting the heart muscle to relax can be one of the biggest challenges we face in treating CHF. Part of the difficulty is often that the heart muscle cells have been replaced by scar tissue. Scar tissue is very stiff, and just like a shirt that has shrunk in the drier, it does not typically stretch back to its normal size and shape. On the other hand, if we relax the heart muscle too much, the heart muscle won't contract forcefully enough to squeeze the blood out of the heart. In this situation, we exchange a problem with the relaxation phase of the heartbeat for a problem with the contraction phase of the heartbeat, but the symptoms do not improve. Getting the heart muscle to relax just the right amount can be a difficult, delicate challenge, so we typically start with small doses of medications and increase them slowly. Also, once a patient is stabilized on a regimen of medications that is adequately relaxing the heart muscle, it's often necessary to adjust the medications periodically as the person's symptoms fluctuate with time. During periods when the heart is not functioning adequately, blood may back up again and there may be an accumulation of fluid in the body. One way many doctors monitor for this fluid accumulation is to have their patients who are being treated for CHF weigh themselves daily. If the patient's weight increases by five pounds or more in a day, the weight gain is most likely due to excessive fluid retention. When this happens, we typically use water pills (called **diuretics**) to help the body get rid of the extra water that has accumulated. Diuretics are usually crucial to the management of CHF. Unfortunately, diuretics put extra strain on the kidneys as they stimulate them to eliminate the extra water, and in the process, the kidneys eliminate electrolytes as well. The most common electrolyte that can be depleted with diuretic use is potassium. For this reason, lab tests need to be run periodically to check potassium levels, and potassium-containing pills or liquids may need to be prescribed in some cases. Electrolyte imbalances and strain on the kidneys make the use of diuretics challenging, but diuretics are a necessary tool in the management of CHF. It can be difficult to balance the beneficial actions of the medications we need with the side effects from these medications. Many physicians manage patients with congestive heart failure, but if a patient's situation is particularly precarious, we may refer that patient to a **cardiologist** (a doctor who specializes in the diagnosis and treatments of abnormalities of the heart) who may take over the management of a more complex case.

It's one problem when the heart muscle can't relax enough to let enough blood into the heart, and it's completely another problem when the heart muscle can't squeeze enough of the blood out of the heart. In this case, the heart fills up with a normal amount of blood, or even more blood than normal, but when the heart muscle tries to squeeze it out, the muscle can't squeeze hard enough. In this situation, the heart muscle is relatively flabby. This flabbiness can occur due to long-term issues that gradually wear the heart out (somewhat like erosion slowly wearing away the soil on a hill), or it can be caused by an event that happens suddenly, stunning the heart (similar to an earthquake suddenly breaking the hill apart). The most common cause of long-term, gradual heart muscle deterioration is high blood pressure (also called **hypertension**). The most common sudden cause of heart muscle weakness is a heart attack (also called a **myocardial infarction**). Another sudden cause of heart muscle injury is an infection with a virus (called **viral myocarditis**). Whatever the cause, the end result is the same...a flabby heart does not pump out enough blood. In order to better understand how a "flabby" heart functions, we need to first look at how a normal heart functions. In a healthy individual, when the heart relaxes, it can fill up with about four ounces of blood. Normally, it will squeeze out about two ounces of this blood with each beat. This means that with an average heart rate of 80 beats per minutes, our hearts pump about 160 ounces (or 1 1/4 gallons) of blood per minute which equals 75 gallons of blood per hour or 1800 gallons of blood per day (pretty impressive if you ask me). This is the amount of blood our various body parts need in order to receive the oxygen and nutrients required to function normally. A flabby heart may only able to squeeze out ½ to 1 ounce of blood with each beat, dropping the daily pumping function to 450-900 gallons per day. While this is still a lot of fluid to pump in a day, it's not enough blood to meet the body's requirements. Just as with diastolic dysfunction, the two problems created with inadequate pumping action of the heart are fluid accumulation in the lungs and inadequate blood flow to the rest of the body. Again, the body needs energy and not pollutants. The end result of low volumes of blood moving through our bodies and leakage of fluid into our lungs is that our bodies feel tired. We call this reduced-pumping type of congestive heart failure **systolic dysfunction (systole** (pronounced sí-stō-lē) is the part of the heart beat when the heart muscle squeezes the blood out of the heart). The treatments for systolic dysfunction are somewhat different than those for diastolic dysfunction. They are focused on increasing the amount of blood the heart pumps out with each beat. To accomplish this, we try to make it easier for the heart to pump the blood into the **arteries** (the blood vessels that carry blood away from the heart) by using blood pressure medications that open the arteries. We also may employ some medications that stimulate the heart to squeeze harder along with diuretics to help the body eliminate the extra water from the lungs. Just as with diastolic dysfunction, management of systolic dysfunction can require a complex, ever-changing combination of medications, and working closely with your doctor is the key to good control of symptoms.

As we touched on earlier, both systolic and diastolic dysfunction can be caused by high blood pressure. Since hypertension is such an important disease among Americans, I will provide a little more detailed description of what hypertension is and how it affects our hearts. Our hearts pump blood into the arteries, and there is some amount of pressure in those arteries at all times (both during systole and during diastole). During systole, our hearts squeeze blood out with a certain amount of force, and the force created inside the heart needs to be greater than the pressure in the arteries in order for the blood to move forward. The measurement of the pressure in the arteries both before and after the heart squeezes blood into them is called **blood pressure.** There are always two numbers reported with a blood pressure (e.g. 120/80). The top number is the maximum amount of pressure the heart creates in the arteries during systole, and we call that number the **systolic blood pressure**. The bottom number is the lowest amount of pressure that remains in the arteries when the heart is relaxing during diastole, and we call that number the **diastolic blood pressure**. A normal blood pressure is 120/80. With a few rare exceptions, blood pressures lower than that are OK, but blood pressures higher than that (and especially higher than 140/90) can cause problems. When the heart is pumping blood against higher-than-normal blood pressure, it needs to work harder than normal in order to push the same amount of blood around the body. The heart is made of muscle. Just like other muscles in the body, the heart can get stronger with increased work, and just like other muscles in the body, when the heart muscle gets stronger, it gets bigger. Unfortunately, while a bigger muscle looks good on the outside of the body, a bigger muscle on the inside of the heart just takes up space, and the space it takes up is space that would otherwise be filled with blood. If the heart muscle becomes too big, there's less room on the inside of the heart for blood to enter the heart, and this creates diastolic dysfunction. On the other side of this analogy, many of us have had the experience of having started a new exercise routine and then having given it up because the workout was too intense. The same thing can happen to the heart. If the blood pressure is too high for the heart, the heart may give up pumping against the increased pressure. When the heart gives up, the patient experiences systolic dysfunction congestive heart failure. Controlling blood pressure is critical for preventing many long-term complications including heart attacks, strokes, and congestive heart failure. Unfortunately, most people with hypertension don't feel the increased pressure in the arteries, and they don't know that damage is being done to the heart and the arteries until it's too late. To compound the problem, most medications used to treat blood pressure have side effects, so when a person takes his blood pressure medications, he may feel worse than he does when he doesn't take his medications. This creates a tricky decision for many patients with hypertension—take my medications and feel bad now or don't take my medications and feel really bad (or die) later. My bias, as a doctor, is to prevent the major long-term problems associated with uncontrolled hypertension, but ultimately, the decision is up to the patient. Some patients take their medications routinely. Some never take their medications. Some only take their medications when they come to my office. I usually tell my patients that ultimately, I'm not the one who needs to know if they're taking their medications, and I'm not the one who has to live with the consequences of not taking them. Ultimately, it's my patient's heart that will know what his blood pressure has been every minute of every day. Again, if you have hypertension, I strongly encourage you to consider taking your medications every day, and if there's a reason you don't take your medications routinely, I encourage you to discuss your concerns with your doctor with the hope that she might help you find better alternatives.

Hypertension means having higher-than-normal pressures in the arteries. A related concept involves the pressure in the arteries being too low. This condition is called **hypotension**. With hypotension, the heart does not squeeze enough blood into the arteries to maintain adequate pressure. This means the amount of blood moving through the arteries will be relatively small, and the body will not receive the amount of oxygen and nutrients it needs. This is like trying to run a sprinkler with the water spigot half opened. The stream coming out of the sprinkler is weak, and there may not be enough pressure to spread water on your lawn. With hypotension, there may not be enough pressure to spread blood around the body. Reduced blood flow is most critical in the brain, and with hypotension, low blood flow into the brain typically causes people to feel dizzy and fatigued. If the blood pressure is relatively normal while lying or sitting but drops when you stand up (again, typically making you feel dizzy or lightheaded as soon as you go from sitting or lying to standing), this is what we call **orthostatic hypotension** (orthostatic means the blood pressure changes when you stand up). The most common cause of orthostatic hypotension is dehydration—less water in the blood causes the total volume of blood to be lower than normal, and a lower total blood volume means there's less blood available for the heart to pump to the rest of the body. Since drinking more fluids will increase the amount of water in the blood, this is the easiest way to treat dehydration and is the easiest way to treat most cases of orthostatic hypotension. The second most common cause of hypotension is as a side effect from medications. A wide variety of medications cause hypotension, and some combinations of medications can worsen symptoms. If you're experiencing hypotension that is causing you to have symptoms (fatigue, dizziness, lightheadedness) and if you've tried increasing your fluid intake without a change in your symptoms, consider reviewing your medications (including your over-the-counter medications and vitamin supplements) with either your doctor or your pharmacist to see if there are changes that can be made to your medication regimen that are likely to improve your hypotension and the associated fatigue.

Besides the pressure that is created in the arteries with each heartbeat, another important part of how the heart functions is the way it's designed to cause the blood to flow in the correct direction. The key to one-way blood flow through the heart is the presence of four one-way valves. In order for these valves to work correctly, they need to open fully and close fully. If any of these valves don't open as much as they are supposed to (we call this situation **stenosis**), less blood is able to flow forward through the heart. This is similar to the decreased shower pressure associated with the reduced water flow through a showerhead that is partially clogged with calcium deposits. Stenosed heart valves lead to low blood flow into the rest of the body, and this can cause many of the symptoms we just discussed relating to hypotension and congestive heart failure. Unfortunately, treating a valvular stenosis isn't easy. In some cases, we can stretch the valve open again (called a **valvuloplasty**). In other cases, it's better to just replace the valve, either with an artificial valve or a valve from a pig's heart. (If you're wondering why we use pig valves, it's because they are similar in size and shape to human valves. The advantage of a pig valve is that it allows for smoother blood flow through it which means that there's a minimal risk of a blood clot forming on the valve. The disadvantage of a pig valve is that it wears out fairly quickly, so it needs to be replaced more often. The advantage of an artificial valve is that it lasts essentially forever. The disadvantage of an artificial valve is that blood clots can form on the valve, so we need to use blood thinner medications to prevent these potential blood clots. Unfortunately, blood thinner medications can be difficult to manage and can lead to unexpected bleeding, so we prefer not to use them if possible.) Finally, for some cases of valvular stenosis, the risks associated with repairing or replacing the valve are too high, and our only option is to try to treat the symptoms the patient is experiencing with medications. As you can tell, valvular stenosis is a complex and very important problem. Your doctor may suspect you have valvular stenosis based on your symptoms. She may also hear noises (that we call **murmurs**) when she listens to your heart. (Incidentally, some people simply have heart murmurs that are a normal part of a normal, healthy heart's functioning, so just because your doctor hears a heart murmur does not mean that something bad or dangerous is going on with your heart.) Ultimately, you will need to have an ultrasound of your heart performed (called an **echocardiogram** or "**echo**" for short) in order to diagnose valvular stenosis. During this echo, we will evaluate which, if any, of the four heart valves are stenosed and how bad the stenoses are. Based on the findings, you will most likely need to be seen by either a **cardiologist** (a doctor who specializes in treating heart conditions) or a **cardiothoracic surgeon** (a doctor who specializes in doing surgery on the heart) to discuss the treatment options available for your case of valvular stenosis.

There can also be problems if the valves don't close all the way (we call this **valvular incompetence** or **valvular regurgitation**). In order for the heart to be effective at pushing the blood through the arteries, the heart needs to push the blood forward with each squeezing of the heart muscle (also called a **contraction**), and the blood that just moved out of the heart has to stay out when the heart muscle relaxes. The primary job of the heart valves is to prevent the blood from reentering the heart during the relaxation of the heart muscle. If these valves don't close all the way and are leaky, they will allow too much of the blood that just left the heart to flow back in again. As more and more blood flows backwards, less and less blood will flow forwards. The result is similar to the problem when the valves don't open enough—the body doesn't get enough blood flowing through it. This can lead to inadequate oxygen and nutrients being brought to the rest of the body, and it can lead to waste products building up. It can also cause congestive heart failure. As we've discussed several times, these circumstances can cause fatigue. The treatments for valvular regurgitation are again very complex. For some abnormalities, surgery and valve repair or replacement can be the best options. For other situations, valve surgery only makes the problem worse, and medications are used. As we discussed with valvular stenosis, an echo will be used to evaluate your heart valve function and potentially make the diagnosis of valvular regurgitation. Once you've been diagnosed with valvular regurgitation, a discussion of treatment options with your cardiologist or your cardiothoracic surgeon will guide your treatment plan. With any heart valve abnormality, ongoing echocardiograms will be very important to monitor the effectiveness of the chosen treatment and to ensure your heart functions at full capacity.

As mentioned above, the heart is like a balloon with the wall of the balloon being made of muscle. Just like other muscles in the body, in order for the heart muscle to perform at peak levels, it needs nutrients and oxygen, too. As odd as it might seem, even though the heart muscle is surrounded by blood, the oxygen and nutrients can't soak into the muscle tissue very well because it's too thick. So, the heart muscle receives blood through its own set of arteries (called **coronary arteries**). If these arteries are blocked (most typically by cholesterol although sugar from diabetes and thickening of the arteries from hypertension and smoking can also cause blockages), not enough blood will flow into the heart muscle. In this situation, the heart muscle itself won't get enough nutrients and oxygen, and the heart will tire more easily than it normally would. This can sometimes cause pain without actually injuring the heart muscle. We call this pain **angina**. Angina is usually associated with chest pain during activity. With angina, the pain goes away with rest. Angina can be a sign that the coronary arteries are becoming dangerously blocked. Any time you suspect you are having the symptoms of angina, it is very important to discuss them with your doctor so he can investigate the cause in more detail. This evaluation will typically involve some sort of **exercise stress test** that is performed by having a person walk on a treadmill while monitoring heart activity. The heart muscle has nerve cells in it, and these nerve cells act as wires carrying electricity from one part of the heart to the others. As the electricity passes through these nerve cells, the muscle tissue in the vicinity contracts.   An organized, coordinated movement of electricity through the heart leads to an organized, coordinated contraction of the muscle, and this allows the heart to actually push the blood out of the heart. Sometimes, when the level of oxygen and nutrients being carried through the coronary is too low, the electricity doesn't move through the heart normally.   The movement of electricity through the heart can be measured using a machine called an **electrocardiograph**. The electrocardiograph senses the electricity moving through the heart and translates the information it gathers onto a piece of paper (the printout is called an **electrocardiogram** or "ECG" or "EKG"). If we're concerned about the possibility of angina, we may start our investigation looking for the disease by performing an exercise stress test. During the test, we attach an electrocardiograph, and we monitor the EKG tracing while the patient exercises. We typically monitor the EKG tracing looking for any changes in the pattern of electricity suggestive of inadequate blood flow into the heart muscle. We commonly combine the EKG monitoring with a type of x-ray that is designed to measure the amount of blood that has entered specific parts of the heart muscle. Both the EKG and the x-ray test are indirect measurements of blood flow into the heart muscle. If there are any suspicious findings during the exercise stress test or on the x-ray test, most cardiologists move on to another diagnostic test that is able to tell exactly which coronary arteries are affected and how large a blockage is present. This next step in evaluating angina is called a cardiac catheterization. During this procedure, the cardiologist is able to put a small tube inside the heart and into the coronary arteries and inject a dye into the various parts of the heart and the different coronary arteries. The cardiologist is then able to see if any portion of the heart is not functioning correctly, and she is able to see how large a blockage, if any, is present in each coronary artery. If a coronary artery blockage is identified, the cardiologist is often able to fix the blockage during the procedure. In general terms, if a blockage is found, the cardiologist may perform an **angioplasty** (a procedure in which a very small, deflated balloon is attached to the end of a wire; the balloon is placed in the center of the blockage (something like putting a piece of thread through the eye of a needle); the balloon is then blown up; and as the balloon expands, it stretches and eventually breaks the blockage). Sometimes, depending on the size and location of the artery being treated, an angioplasty works well enough to produce a long-lasting open artery. Sometimes, the artery has a tendency to shrink back down to the pre-angioplasty size.   In the latter case, a stent (which is a metal tube that is something like a spring that can be compressed to fit into a smaller space and that opens up into a full-sized tube when it is released) is placed in the part of an artery where an angioplasty has just been performed as a means of trying to keep the coronary artery open. Angina is a warning sign that a significant blockage of a coronary artery is developing, and the minimally-invasive techniques used to diagnose and treat these blockages save thousands of lives every year. If you suspect you have angina, don't delay seeing your doctor to discuss your symptoms and any additional testing you will require to identify your potential problem.

Angina is a transient condition associated with short periods of time during which segments of heart muscle temporarily do not get enough blood flow. If, instead, blood stops flowing completely to a segment of heart muscle for a prolonged period of time, the part of the heart muscle that is no longer receiving blood flow can die, and this is what we refer to as a heart attack or a **myocardial infarction (MI))**. If a patient who is experiencing the early stages of an MI immediately calls emergency services and is quickly treated in an emergency room, the heart muscle that is beginning to die can be saved. If there is a delay in opening a blocked coronary artery, more and more of the heart muscle will continue to die. The longer the delay, the larger the area of heart muscle that is killed. If the damage is severe, the remaining heart muscle may be insufficient to pump blood adequately to the rest of the body. As we discussed earlier, less blood flow through the body equals less nutrients and more waste. This leads to our feeling fatigued. Since heart attacks are the leading cause of death in the United States, maintaining good heart health is a primary goal for most doctors, and controlling blood pressure, diabetes, and cholesterol levels are our main focus in preventing heart attacks. In order to prevent heart attacks, patients also need to take an active role in managing their medical conditions. If you or someone you know begins to experience symptoms that might be related to a heart attack, the sooner you're seen and treated by a doctor, the better chance you have of saving as much heart muscle as possible.

The final circulatory issue I will discuss does not involve the heart or the blood vessels but rather involves the blood itself. As we've discussed several times, two of the primary functions of our blood are to transport oxygen and nutrients to the places they are needed and then to return the waste products to the places where they are eliminated. If the blood does not perform these tasks correctly, our bodies will run out of energy, and waste products will build up. In order to carry around enough nutrients, there has to be enough blood. If the total amount of blood in your body is low, you will feel fatigued. If this is the case, you will typically, but not always, have orthostatic hypotension as described above. You may also show signs of **dehydration** (which include decreased urination, dark yellow or brown urine, feeling fatigued, feeling achy, having a headache, and possibly feeling nauseated). Most of these symptoms are only experienced with a sudden drop in blood volume. When the drop in blood volume is slow and gradual, fatigue may be your only symptom. If you are suspicious that you might be dehydrated, the best first step you can take at home is to increase your fluid intake (especially with fluids containing electrolytes like sports drinks). If increased fluid intake improves your fatigue, continuing to drink a larger volume of fluids on a daily basis will likely prevent future episodes of symptomatic dehydration. If increased fluid intake doesn't improve your symptoms, keep searching for the cause.

It's also possible to feel fatigued and to have enough blood volume but to not have enough of certain components of the blood. There are various components of blood that perform different functions, and if these functions are not being performed correctly, you will feel fatigued. In order to figure out if you have specific problems with your blood, your doctor will need to perform a few simple lab tests that we will discuss briefly now and in more detail in the next chapter. Our blood is made up of many components, but for our discussion here, I want to focus on two of the most important. These are the oxygen-carrying component, **hemoglobin**, and the nutrient-carrying component, **serum**. We often think of hemoglobin as a bunch of boxcars in a train that has the job of transporting oxygen from the lungs (where oxygen levels are the highest) to the rest of our bodies (where the oxygen levels are lower). Without enough hemoglobin, there aren't enough boxcars to carry the oxygen to the needy tissues, and the tissues run out of energy. A low level of hemoglobin is called **anemia**. Anemia can have several causes, the most common of which is inadequate iron intake through our diets. Iron is one of the key building blocks of hemoglobin, and if we do not eat enough iron on a daily basis, hemoglobin cannot be manufactured in adequate quantities by our bodies. Taking iron supplements can help with many causes of anemia, but much of the iron taken in through supplements is not absorbed by the intestines. There are some forms of iron supplements that are absorbed better by our intestines than others. Discussing with your pharmacist the iron supplements available at your pharmacy, and reviewing with your pharmacist the ways to improve iron absorption is the best way to help you choose the correct supplement for you so you can effectively treat iron deficiency anemia once it's diagnosed by your doctor. Iron is the key chemical needed to make hemoglobin, and hemoglobin production begins when our kidneys sense that our hemoglobin levels are too low. In response to low levels of hemoglobin, our kidneys release a hormone, called **erythropoietin**, which sends a signal to our **bone marrow** (the soft center portion inside of some of our bones) to produce more **red blood cells (RBCs)** (the cells in the blood that contain hemoglobin). This process of producing more RBCs along with the other cells in the blood is called **hematopoiesis**. If the kidneys are unable, or unwilling, to produce enough erythropoietin or if our bone marrow doesn't respond appropriately to the erythropoietin that's produced, anemia can develop.   When anemia develops, again, there aren't enough boxcars to carry enough oxygen to all the parts of the body and the person will feel fatigued. Unlike treating iron-deficiency anemia, the form of anemia caused by not producing enough red blood cells (called **aplastic anemia**) is more difficult to diagnose and treat. The diagnosis is typically made through a combination of blood testing and a biopsy of the bone marrow. Depending on the findings of these tests, the treatments also require you to work closely with your doctor over time to repair and maintain adequate RBC and hemoglobin levels. This is a complicated disease with many treatable and some non-treatable causes, and most patients will work with a **hematologist/oncologist** (a doctor who specializes in diagnosing and treating medical problems of the blood (**hematology**) as well as diagnosing and treating cancers (**oncology**)) when looking for a successful treatment for aplastic anemia.

While aplastic anemia is the result of the body not making enough red blood cells, another, somewhat similar, form of anemia results when the body makes a normal number of RBCs and they are then prematurely destroyed. A normal red blood cell circulates through our bodies for about four months. After completing their four-month journey, the worn out red blood cells are filtered out and destroyed by our **spleens** (the spleen is an organ in the body that is responsible for filtering out used RBCs as well as filtering out certain kinds of infections from the blood). When a red blood cell is destroyed, a portion of the hemoglobin is recycled back into a new red blood cell. Occasionally, due to abnormally-shaped red blood cells or due to an overactive filtering system in the spleen, red blood cells are destroyed more frequently than every four months. Since only a portion of the hemoglobin contained in each red blood cell is recycled, some of the extra hemoglobin is excreted either in the urine or the feces. As more and more of the hemoglobin is excreted, the hemoglobin levels slowly fall to the point where we develop iron deficiency anemia. We call the premature destruction of RBCs leading to anemia **hemolytic anemia**, and as with aplastic anemia, the causes and treatments of hemolytic anemia are very complicated. Working closely with your doctor (and most likely a hematologist/oncologist) and discussing different medications and possible surgery will be necessary to manage it successfully.

The other component of blood we will discuss in this section of the book is the serum. **Serum** is essentially the watery part of blood in which all the rest of the nutrients are dissolved. Serum makes up about 2/3 of the volume of the blood that circulates through our bodies. Consisting primarily of water, serum levels can drop significantly if we become dehydrated. Most of the rest of our bodies are made up of water as well, and we are dependent on maintaining adequate water levels within our bodies in order for our bodies to function normally. Drinking and eating are our only means of bringing water into our bodies. We lose water in many ways, including in our urine, in our stool, in our sweat, and in our breath as we exhale. Through extensive research, we have come to understand exactly how much **water we lose each day**, and from this we can calculate the amount of water we need to take in for an average day. This number can change significantly if we change any of the variables used to determine the baseline number (for example if we are exercising and are breathing more quickly and sweating more than usual, our water intake will need to be increased; if we are experiencing diarrhea causing us to lose extra water into our stool, our water intake will need to be increased; or if we are on water pills causing us to lose extra water into our urine, our water intake will need to be increased as well.) At baseline, the amount of water we need to take in is based on our weight, and the formula is as follows: for the first 100 pounds of a person's weight, he must drink roughly 35 ½ ounces (about 4 ½ cups) of water per day to maintain his fluid balance. For each 10 pounds above the first 100 pounds, he would need to drink about two more ounces of water per day. So, for a person who weighs 170 pounds, for example, we would figure his baseline daily water intake requirement as follows: 35 ½ ounces (for the first 100 pounds) plus 14 ounces (2 ounces for each of the 7 sets of 10 pounds above 100 pounds). This person needs to drink a minimum of approximately 49 ½ ounces (a little more than six cups) of water per day in order to maintain a stable amount of water in his body at baseline (i.e. minimal activity and no significant sweating, vomiting, or diarrhea). Some of this water can come from beverages, and some of it can come from foods (water content in any particular food is a little more difficult to guestimate, so you'll have to take your best stab when trying to work that into the equation.) Beware! Caffeine and alcohol act as **diuretics** (they cause our kidneys to put out extra water), so drinking four cans of caffeine-containing, diet soda or four beers actually counts as a negative when keeping track of the number of cups of water taken in each day. This means you might need to drink seven or eight cups of water on top of the caffeinated sodas or alcohol just to meet your basic requirements. If you happen to exercise or do any kind of a physical job that causes you to sweat or breathe heavily, you will need to add to the baseline six cups you need each day. If we do not maintain adequate fluid intake, we will become dehydrated fairly quickly. Dehydration translates into a decreased total serum volume. Since serum makes up the majority of the volume of our blood, a decreased serum level means that there will be a decreased total blood volume. When the total blood volume is low, there is less blood for the heart to circulate. This causes inadequate blood flow to the rest of the body that causes insufficient supply of energy and incomplete removal of waste products, and we go on to suffer the complications of dehydration as described above.

Understanding that we all have busy lives and may not be able to keep an exact tally on the precise number of ounces of water we drink each day and understanding that our activity levels vary greatly each day, as does the amount of water in the foods we eat from day to day, it's not reasonable to try to calculate the "correct" amount of water you need to drink each day down to the

51

very ounce. The numbers I gave above are just starting points. With that in mind, we must acknowledge that most of the time we'll either drink too much water or not enough water on any given day. Knowing that drinking too little water can cause dehydration that causes a variety of undesirable symptoms, it's much better to err on the side of drinking too much water each day. Luckily for most of us, we have normal kidneys that are amazing organs. Normal kidneys are able to take in water and various electrolytes, keep what they need, and get rid of what they don't need. That means that, as a general rule, we can drink plenty of extra water and electrolytes, and our kidneys will be smart enough to keep what they need and get rid of the excess. It is possible to overrun our kidneys, and I'm sure we all remember the story about the radio contest in California back in 2007 that led to a woman drinking a large amount of water that led to her death. She died from something called **water intoxication** that is caused by drinking a very large amount of water (something along the lines of two gallons) in a very short amount of time (something like one hour). Water intoxication is a problem because the kidneys aren't able to get rid of the excess water quickly enough. The extra water mixes with the electrolytes in the blood and **dilutes** (or waters down) the electrolytes. Correct levels of all of the electrolytes are important, but water intoxication is most crucial in regards to sodium. With water intoxication, the sodium becomes significantly diluted, and the level of sodium throughout the body becomes too low. Low levels of sodium in the body are referred to as **hyponatremia**, and with rapid development of hyponatremia, a life-threatening situation can occur. Luckily it's rare to overwhelm normal kidneys' ability to regulate water and electrolyte levels. As a rule, if we drink a cup or two of water every hour or two, our kidneys should be able to get rid of the excess water without any problems. The same applies to other electrolytes. Even if we take in extra amounts of sodium or potassium or calcium, our kidneys should be able to get rid of the excess. This, of course, is only true for normal kidneys. In general, people with hypertension or diabetes cannot be assumed to have normal kidney function. Additionally, over time our kidneys age and their function declines, so the older we get, the less flexible our kidneys become. This means that, if you are young and healthy, you can feel comfortable gradually increasing, over a week's time, your daily fluid intake from six cups (48 ounces) of water spread throughout each day to a gallon (148 ounces) of water spread throughout each day. A gallon of water intake each day should be enough for all but the heaviest sweaters or the people with the worst cases of vomiting and diarrhea, so it's a good goal for most people. If you have any concerns about your medical conditions or how well your kidneys are functioning and how well they will handle extra water and electrolyte intake, performing lab tests is the only way to know for sure where you stand.   This means that you will need to schedule an appointment with your doctor to have the lab tests performed and to discuss the results of the tests with her. Once you have the lab test results, you can discuss the option of increased water intake with her as well.

We've spent a lot of time reviewing circulatory complications because they are frequent causes of fatigue. Our bodies are resilient and can compensate for many deviations from their normal states, but if a particular strain becomes severe enough, our bodies will stop functioning properly.   Proper functioning is dependent on our circulatory systems obtaining oxygen and nutrients in adequate levels and removing waste products efficiently. When there is inadequate circulation, a deficit of oxygen or other nutrients develops, and waste products accumulate. Eventually, once the level of circulatory insufficiency reaches a certain point, we realize that we don't have the energy we used to have. This is when we start to recognize that something is not right with our bodies.   Some circulatory issues can be identified and treated at home, but most require a discussion with your doctor. Pay attention to what your body is telling you. As soon as you feel like you don't have the energy you used to have, start to take some of the corrective steps described above. If those actions don't improve the way you feel, don't hesitate to schedule an appointment with your doctor.

Chapter 4: Causes of Fatigue—Body Chemistry

So far, we've discussed the two most common categories of fatigue-causing disorders. In the next couple chapters, I will round out the picture of the remaining problems that steal energy away from my patients. Our bodies are very complex, and there are many different individual systems that interact with each other in order to keep the whole body functioning normally. This interaction almost always represents a delicate balance between one system trying to push things in one direction and another system trying to push things in the opposite direction. It's like trying to balance on a balance beam. If we feel ourselves starting to fall off the beam to the left, our tendency is to lean to the right. But leaning too far to the right can cause us to start to fall to the right, so we lean back to the left. It's the constant struggle between leaning to the left and leaning to the right that (hopefully) keeps us balanced on the beam. To this point, we have discussed a few of the ways our bodies maintain this balance in order to continue to function normally. This balance is important, even down to the sub-microscopic level. Inside our bodies there are thousands of chemicals, each one performing a very specific job. The chemicals work in conjunction with each other to accomplish a variety of goals. If one chemical in the mix is not present or does not function properly, the entire balancing act will fail, and our bodies will experience the consequences. In general, our bodies are very adept at maintaining the proper levels of all the chemicals and ensuring they all function properly, but occasionally, one of the chemicals gets out of balance and problems ensue. In this chapter, I will discuss the most important chemicals that, when out of balance, cause fatigue. I will explain what functions these chemicals perform in our bodies as well as what happens when they aren't performing their functions correctly.

As mentioned in the previous chapter, oxygen is one of the most important chemicals to our bodies. **Oxygen** is one of the primary sources of energy that allows the different parts of our bodies to perform their normal functions. We've already discussed what happens when there isn't enough oxygen brought to our tissues due to circulatory problems, but now I'll discuss some other reasons oxygen levels can drop below normal. Oxygen enters the blood stream through the lungs. As we discussed before, the spaces within the lungs contain air (21% of which is oxygen), and the solid portions of the lungs contain blood. We call one of these air spaces surrounded by the solid portion an **alveous** (plural is **alveoli**). These alveoli allow the oxygen to enter the blood from the air and, at the same time, allow the carbon dioxide to exit the blood back into the air. The walls of the alveoli are very thin and fragile. If they are destroyed or if they are thickened, oxygen and carbon dioxide have a harder time passing from the air into the blood and vice versa. The next group of fatigue-causing disorders we will discuss will be those that affect the function of the alveoli.

The most common cause of destruction of these fragile alveoli is cigarette smoking. Smoke of any kind is very irritating and even toxic to the lung cells. Each puff of smoke kills off a handful of cells. Fortunately, our lungs are able to compensate for this damage—at least for a while. Eventually, however, when enough alveoli have been destroyed, an imbalance arises between the amount of blood flowing through the lungs and the number of places the blood can stop to pick up oxygen and drop off carbon dioxide. If we use the boxcar analogy from the last chapter, there become fewer train stations present in the lungs which means the trains have fewer places to stop to pick up oxygen and drop off carbon dioxide. This means that fewer boxcars are able to fill up and empty out with each pass through the lungs. Instead of 99 or 100% of the boxcars filling with oxygen, now only 85 or 90% are able to fill up. With continued smoking, this number decreases even further. As there are fewer boxcars filled with oxygen and more filled with carbon dioxide, less oxygen is passed to the tissues that need it, and more carbon dioxide builds up in these tissues.   Through the chain of events described earlier, we feel fatigued.

As long as we're discussing smoking and the hemoglobin boxcars, I'd like to mention one other passenger that rides the hemoglobin train.   This passenger is carbon monoxide.   As discussed earlier, carbon monoxide is produced whenever something, including tobacco, is burned. Carbon monoxide likes to fill places on hemoglobin, just like oxygen.   Unfortunately, carbon monoxide will often remain permanently stuck to hemoglobin until the red blood cell is destroyed. Since carbon monoxide is taking up space on the hemoglobin train, there's less room for oxygen to stick to the same hemoglobin. This translates into fewer boxcars available to carry oxygen within our bodies. Having fewer boxcars carrying oxygen means we end up with a problem similar to anemia. Symptoms that are associated with **carbon monoxide poisoning** (nausea, headache, and sleepiness) occur when there's an exposure to a large, sudden dose of carbon monoxide (the furnace vent pipe gets plugged up, and you wake up in the morning feeling sick). Unfortunately, long-term exposure to carbon monoxide, like we see in smokers, typically does not cause dramatic symptoms, and many long-term smokers may not feel sick at all (except for some possible fatigue) because the carbon monoxide poisoning has happened so gradually. It's something like gaining weight.   If you gain 10 pounds in a week on a vacation, you (and probably everyone around you) will likely notice the extra puffiness in your midsection. If, instead, you gain the same 10 pounds gradually over a year, you are less likely to notice the change until you realize your pants don't fit like they used to. With smoking, you may not feel the effects until several years later when you notice that you're fatigued and that your exercise tolerance has dropped. Since there are very few other causes of chronic carbon monoxide poisoning besides smoking, quitting smoking (and/or not spending time around people who are smoking, since second-hand smoke has many of the same effects and complications as smoking the cigarettes yourself) is the best way to fix this common cause of fatigue. Anyone who has tried to quit smoking can tell you how difficult it is. Nicotine is one of the most addictive drugs known to man. Later in the book, I will discuss some of the methods commonly used to help quit smoking. For now, the most important thing is to recognize that quitting smoking is very helpful with improving many medical conditions, including fatigue.

Another injury we can cause to the alveoli is increasing their wall thickness. Normally, the walls of our alveoli are extremely thin, allowing for easy passage of oxygen and carbon dioxide through them. If these walls become thickened, usually due to chronic irritation or "inflammation," oxygen and carbon dioxide cannot cross as easily. **Inflammation** is the body's response to irritation. When a part of the body is irritated, there's a cascade of different chemicals (called **inflammatory mediators**) that's released. The purpose of these mediators is to stimulate the body's immune system to get rid of the thing that is causing the irritation. Unfortunately, sometimes the inflammatory mediators cause unintended side effects. Chronic inflammation of the lungs, for example, causes thickening and even scarring of the walls of the alveoli that can lead to poor oxygen and carbon dioxide movement into and out of the body. There are several causes of chronic inflammation of the alveoli, among which is asthma. **Asthma** is defined as inflammation of the air tubes in the lungs as well as of the alveoli. The symptoms of an **acute asthma exacerbation** are coughing, wheezing, feeling short of breath, and a decrease in exercise tolerance. Unfortunately the lung injury associated with **chronic asthma** may not create any noticeable symptoms. For this reason, periodic breathing tests at your doctor's office (called **pulmonary function testing**) or at your home (called **peek flow testing**) are often used to monitor the status and progression of asthma. There's a variety of causes of the inflammation associated with asthma including exposure to chemicals that stimulate allergic reactions (things like pollen, dust, pet dander, smoke, and perfume) as well as respiratory illnesses, exercise, and exposure to cold temperatures. Asthma is often inherited from our parents, although this pattern can be difficult to identify because asthma symptoms were commonly overlooked or ignored in the past. For this reason, many adults have experienced asthma symptoms but have never been diagnosed with asthma, so there is no clear family history of it. If someone is diagnosed with asthma, he is usually treated for the disease. Treatments for asthma include a variety of inhalers or "puffers" to control acute asthma symptoms, along with other inhalers and oral medications to reduce long-term inflammation. Ultimately, our goal for managing asthma is to reduce or eliminate acute asthma flare-ups, as well as to control the long-term inflammation. If we do not gain adequate control of the chronic inflammation component, people with asthma can develop thickening of the walls of their alveoli that can lead to lower oxygen levels and higher carbon dioxide levels in the blood. This is most important when a person suffers with poorly-controlled asthma for many years. This is the main reason it's particularly important to diagnose and control asthma as early in the disease course as possible, especially in children. Undiagnosed or poorly-controlled asthma poses a number of potential problems for children. It may prevent them from participating in certain activities with the rest of their classmates (which can be harmful socially), and the chronic inflammation can also lead to reduced growth rates and shorter adult heights compared to those children who don't suffer from asthma. Again, in order to prevent complications associated with asthma, it's important to control both the acute flare ups and the chronic inflammation. Close monitoring and management of asthma is the key, not only to keeping people with asthma out of the hospital but also to helping them live normal lives and preventing long-term complications. For these reasons, people who have asthma need to fully understand how asthma works, what the symptoms of asthma are, how to monitor for asthma flares even in the absence of significant asthma symptoms, and how to use their asthma medications correctly. This level of understanding only comes with spending extra time learning about these topics from their doctors as well as from asthma educators, pharmacists, and educational materials. If you have been diagnosed with asthma, or if you suspect you have asthma but have not yet been diagnosed with it, be sure to seek out all the educational resources you can find. Even if you've had asthma for many years, the strategies used to monitor and treat asthma are constantly evolving, so reviewing these topics with your doctor on a regular basis is a good idea.

Another equally important chemical, which is the primary fuel source for all our tissues, is **glucose**. Our bodies prefer glucose as a fuel over other forms of calories, and regardless of the form in which energy enters our bodies (fat, protein, or carbohydrates), it's usually converted into glucose before it's used. There's an elaborate network of **enzymes** (which are proteins that perform various jobs) that process most foods and convert them into glucose. Our bodies then either use the glucose directly or convert it into other chemicals (mostly fat) for storage. We have several organs that are involved in the digestion of food and the processing of glucose. The **pancreas** (one of the organs in the abdomen) is the most important organ for glucose control. It senses how much glucose has been taken in during a meal, and in response, it releases an appropriate amount of **insulin** (which is a hormone that allows the glucose to get into the cells of the body). (**Cells** are the building blocks of the body just like individual bricks are the building blocks of a house, and it's the cells of the body that work together to perform the various functions necessary to stay alive.) Insulin circulates with glucose through the blood. While in circulation, some of the glucose and some of the insulin "land" on the cells in need of energy. The insulin acts like a key that opens a doorway into the cell. Once the door is open, a certain amount of the glucose can enter the cell before the door automatically closes again. The glucose that enters the cell while the door is open is the fuel the cell uses to perform its function within the body. If an inadequate amount of glucose enters the cell, the cell won't be able to perform its assigned task. If this happens, the cell will begin to starve, with the most active cells (most importantly the cells in the brain and the cells in the heart) starving first. In order for this glucose/insulin mechanism to work correctly, the system must be very accurate, and the amount of insulin released must be in exact proportion to the amount of glucose present. If too much insulin is released, too much sugar will go into the cells all at once, leaving too little glucose in the blood for future use. This is like going grocery shopping on Sunday and eating all the food you just bought by Monday. By Wednesday, you're pretty hungry. If the cells use all the available glucose immediately (because the extra insulin allowed all the glucose to enter immediately), the blood glucose levels will drop below normal, and the cells will have a harder and harder time functioning correctly. This can lead to extreme fatigue and can even be life threatening. Conversely, if too little insulin is released, the glucose will remain in the blood and not enough will enter the cells. In this case, the cells will run out of fuel, and they will start to starve, even though there's plenty of "food" surrounding them. Again, it's the balance between glucose and insulin that's most important. If there is too much or too little of one or the other component, our cells, and therefore our whole bodies, will experience problems.

When the amount of sugar floating around in the blood is too high, we call this **diabetes mellitus** or just "**diabetes.**" There are two kinds of diabetes. If the pancreas doesn't release enough insulin, this is called **insulin-dependent diabetes mellitus (IDDM)** or **type I diabetes mellitus**. Type I diabetes is identified on blood tests when we find excess glucose present in the blood with very low or absent levels of insulin present. In this scenario, there simply aren't enough keys to open the doors of the cells and let the glucose in. The cells end up running on inadequate supplies of fuel, and their function deteriorates with time. Alternatively, the pancreas can release the correct amount of insulin, but the cells can be resistant to it. These cells have what I describe as "sticky locks." This means that the proper amount of insulin does not open the correct number of doorways. The significance of sticky locks is that, even though there's plenty of insulin in the blood and excess glucose in the blood, the cells still run low on fuel. We refer to this type of diabetes as **non-insulin-dependent diabetes mellitus (NIDDM)** or **type II diabetes mellitus**. Again, the result

61

is that the cells cannot function normally because not enough glucose is getting into them.

Regardless of which type of diabetes a person has, there is an excessive amount of glucose circulating in the blood, but the cells cannot access the fuel source. The cells cannot perform their designated tasks without enough glucose, and they begin to function inefficiently. To compound the problem, the extra glucose from the blood frequently spills out through the urine, carrying water with it. This excess water loss through the kidneys quickly leads to dehydration, and this combination of inadequate glucose usage by the cells along with dehydration can, in extreme cases, lead to a profound, and often disabling, degree of fatigue. Having a blood test done is the only way to tell if your blood glucose levels are too high. The level of glucose in the blood that "defines" diabetes changes periodically, and the timing of the blood test (fasting for eight hours or at a random time or immediately after eating or drinking a certain amount of glucose) also changes in time. If you have any concerns about the possibility that you have diabetes, be sure to discuss your concerns with your doctor so the correct blood test can be run and the correct interpretation can be used to make the diagnosis.

There are many things we know about diabetes, and one of the most important is that the longer a person has diabetes, the more likely he is to develop complications. I always compare the excess glucose molecules circulating around in the blood to hairs that are going through a shower drain. As most people have seen when they clean out a shower drain, a few hairs always seem to get caught on the entry to the drain. At first, the water keeps flowing down the drain, but eventually, the water doesn't flow down the drain anymore. Even though the hair builds up gradually over months or years, most people don't notice it until the water stops draining and there's a big glob of hair completely blocking the drain. With diabetes, the extra glucose molecules stick to parts of the arteries. In time, more and more glucose molecules stick to each other in the arteries. People usually don't notice this is occurring until there's a big glob of glucose molecules blocking blood flow through an artery. By the time you realize you have a problem (whether you first notice a loss of vision or a loss of kidney function or a loss of sensation in your toes or an uncontrolled infection in your foot), it's too late. Unlike removing a mass of hair from a shower drain, we don't have a way to deal with the glob of glucose molecules. This means that once the damage of diabetes is noticed, the damage is permanent. This is the reason diagnosing diabetes early and maintaining good control of the disease is so important. And this is why, if you suspect you might have diabetes, getting in to see your doctor sooner rather than later is so important. Working closely with your doctor, your diabetes educator, your pharmacist, and any other support group in your area to maintain good control of your diabetes is critical.

The energy our bodies use is generated as we burn glucose. We provide our bodies with glucose through the food we eat. Unfortunately, the chemical reactions that convert food into glucose take time which means there can be a delay between when we eat and when the glucose is available for use in our blood. This means that we may run low on glucose while we're waiting for the food we just ate to be turned into glucose. Besides the food we eat, we also have energy reserves. Some of these reserves are in the form of fat stores, and some of the reserves are in another storage form in our livers (called **glycogen** which we will discuss in a moment). If the glucose levels in our blood start to drop, we start converting our energy reserves to glucose. This conversion process from the stored forms of energy to glucose also takes time. Our blood glucose levels can drop significantly while we're waiting for these conversion processes to occur. Having a low blood glucose level is a condition we refer to as **hypoglycemia**. Running low on glucose, which means running low on usable energy, slows down the various functions of the body and leads to fatigue. Hypoglycemia occurs in two basic circumstances—when our pancreases malfunction and when our bodies are burning glucose more rapidly than normal. We will now review both these potential causes of fatigue in more detail.

A malfunction of the pancreas can lead to excessive insulin levels. Excessive insulin levels are the most common and the most dangerous cause of hypoglycemia. Earlier, we discussed the pancreas's role in diabetes—the pancreas's job is to release an amount of insulin that exactly matches the amount of glucose in the bloodstream. Sometimes, the pancreas over responds to a certain glucose level, releasing too much insulin and causing the glucose level to drop too far. This causes hypoglycemia. While hypoglycemia can be caused by the pancreas releasing too much insulin on its own, it's more commonly seen when patients who are being treated for diabetes take too much of their medications. In these situations, the glucose levels can drop significantly, and this can cause severe hypoglycemia which is dangerous and can even be life threatening. Because this can occur in anyone who has diabetes and is taking certain medications for it (ask your doctor or pharmacist if the medications you are taking can cause hypoglycemia), these people should have an emergency form of glucose immediately available. (Glucose is sold as tablets, gel, and liquid. It is important to understand that glucose tablets are NOT the same as hard candy which has **sucrose** that is the form of sugar found in table sugar and that needs to be "digested" into glucose before it can be used by our bodies. Also, glucose liquid is NOT the same as fruit juice which has **fructose** in it that's the form of sugar found in fruits that also needs to be "digested" into glucose before it can be used by our bodies.) If a person who is on medications for diabetes develops symptoms of hypoglycemia (the most common symptoms are fatigue, jitters, nausea, sweating, and confusion) she should check her blood sugar immediately, if possible, and she should take a glucose supplement immediately if the blood sugar is too low. A delay in treatment for severe hypoglycemia can be life-threatening. For this reason, it is critically important for a person who is on medications for diabetes to have a functioning **glucometer** (a machine that measures the amount of glucose in the blood), all the necessary blood glucose testing supplies, and a form of oral glucose readily available in case of an emergency. Diagnosing hypoglycemia requires immediate blood glucose testing when symptoms occur.

Preventing hypoglycemia in patients with diabetes primarily involves carefully adjusting the medications known to cause hypoglycemia with the ultimate goal of lowering the blood glucose levels to a normal level and not below that level. This process can be a delicate balance, and it can take time. This balance can also be thrown off by the foods we eat, changes in weight, daily exercise levels, and the timing and quantity of the diabetes medications taken. For these reasons, if you have concerns about your diabetes medications, be sure to discuss your concerns with your doctor and review your options for changing your medications with her.

I want to review one more key component of blood glucose regulation in our bodies. Besides being able to detect elevated blood glucose levels, the pancreas can also sense low blood glucose levels as well. As the blood glucose approaches this lower threshold, the pancreas releases a hormone called **glucagon** that stimulates our fat cells to convert fat into glucose. It also stimulates our livers to release their storage form of energy (our livers store energy in the form of a chemical called **glycogen** that's like a stack of glucose molecules all clumped together). However, there can be a significant time delay between when the glucose level drops, when the signal to release more glucose is sent from the pancreas, and when the storage form of energy is "digested" releasing an adequate amount of new glucose into the bloodstream. Therefore, in people who use glucose more rapidly or who have inadequate energy storage levels, their blood glucose levels can fall to lower-than-normal levels which deprives their bodies of energy, causing them to feel fatigued. In this situation, the diagnosis of hypoglycemia can be difficult to make. We normally want to be able to measure a blood glucose level at the time when symptoms develop. Since having a blood test done at exactly the correct moment can be difficult to coordinate, most patients have a hard time documenting the low blood sugar if it is happening. In some instances, we may try a variety of different methods to "catch" the hypoglycemia when it shows up. For most folks who are not on diabetes medications, occasional episodes of hypoglycemia are not dangerous, so measuring the low blood sugar with a test isn't always critical. Often times, if you suspect you are having episodes of hypoglycemia, eating smaller meals (which will not trigger as large a release of insulin) and eating them more frequently (six to eight small meals each day) can eliminate the symptoms that can be so bothersome, and this may be the best long-term solution for your fatigue. If adjusting your eating habits doesn't correct the symptoms you suspect are related to hypoglycemia, discuss with your doctor the option of your purchasing a glucometer so an immediate blood glucose measurement can be performed with the presentation of your symptoms. If you find that you are developing episodes of hypoglycemia, discuss the treatment options with your doctor.

Another situation in which our bodies use too much glucose occurs when our metabolism is running at a higher-than-normal rate. Consuming energy too rapidly, our bodies in this overactive state can eventually use up all the energy available to them. Our bodies are built for survival, so they'll start to break down our fat stores in an effort to get enough energy to stay alive. Eventually, they'll even start to break down muscle and use the muscle as a source of energy, but it's difficult for our bodies to break down fat and muscle fast enough to keep up with the energy demands of these overactive states. When our bodies are running out of energy and are struggling to stay alive, many symptoms develop. A person who is running out of energy will often feel achy and possibly nauseated, and they'll typically experience an intense sense of fatigue, or more likely total exhaustion. Such overactive states exist with a variety of different medical conditions. One of these is the situation in which cells begin to grow out of control. This is what we call **cancer**. Cells that are functioning normally in the body have very specific roles, and they operate under very strict controls. Cells typically start and stay in one location, and they have a lifespan. Most cells respond in defined ways to different hormones and other regulatory systems designed to control the cells' functions. Unlike normal cells, cancer cells do not respond to these controls, and as they grow, they can get more and more out of control. They use energy without performing their correct functions. They live long past their defined lifespans. They grow into and move into places they should not go. As there are more and more of these out-of-control cells in the body, they steal more and more energy from the normal cells. This excessive energy use, along with the release of inflammatory mediators that usually accompanies our bodies' attempt to fight the cancer, typically leave a person with cancer feeling exhausted. Clearly, most fatigue is the result of a medical condition other than cancer, and diagnosing and treating cancer are very complicated tasks, especially if the only symptom a patient has is fatigue. Because of the wide variety of cancers that exist and because there are many fatigue-causing disorders that are much more common than cancer, it doesn't make sense to screen every person with fatigue for every kind of cancer. For this reason, there are certain cancers we screen for at different ages for men and for women, and these screening tests are scheduled with the purpose of identifying cancers in the earliest treatable stages with the goal of saving lives. Unfortunately, no cancer screening test is perfectly accurate, and every follow-up diagnostic test and cancer treatment has side effects. For this reason, before we perform a cancer screening test, we always need to weigh the risks and the side effects of the diagnostic tests and treatments against the benefits of finding the cancer at an early stage. Sometimes the benefits are greater, so we recommend performing the screening tests. Sometime the risks are greater, so we recommend not performing the screening tests. The risks, benefits, and recommendations for various cancer screening tests change all the time as new studies are done and new tests are developed. For this reason, it's very important to discuss age-appropriate cancer screening with your doctor annually, even if you are feeling well, and it's even more important to review these screening tests with her if you feel fatigued.

Another hormone that controls how our bodies use energy is called **thyroid hormone**, and it controls even more phases of energy production and utilization than does insulin. Thyroid hormone enters our cells and stimulates them to increase their usage of both glucose and oxygen. It also makes them more sensitive to the effects of adrenaline. This means that, if the level of thyroid hormone is lower than normal (called **hypothyroidism**), the body's metabolism will slow down, and it will use less glucose and less oxygen and subsequently produce less energy within the cells. Also, if the thyroid hormone levels are too low, the heart and brain won't respond to adrenaline like they normally would, and the ability to exercise, as well as mental alertness, will decline. Again, this constellation of symptoms is often conveyed to me by my patients with the word "fatigue." People with hypothyroidism are tired. Thyroid hormone controls the functioning of almost every part of our bodies which means that almost any kind of abnormality in bodily function (from fatigue to weight gain to skin texture changes to constipation to heart palpitations) can be caused by thyroid dysfunction.

Problems can also arise when thyroid hormone levels are too high (called **hyperthyroidism**). As you might imagine, increased levels of thyroid hormone cause increased energy usage by our bodies. When we use too much energy, we have a hard time sleeping. We have a hard time slowing our minds down enough to think clearly. Our hearts may race. We may lose weight unexpectedly. We may become very sweaty, and we may experience anxiety. This constant state of "excitement" can be exhausting, and my patients with hyperthyroidism frequently experience "fatigue," too.

Whether our thyroid hormone levels are too low or too high, we don't feel like ourselves. Luckily, there are simple blood tests doctors use to identify low or high thyroid hormone levels. Depending on whether the hormone levels are high or low, the treatments involved can be relatively simple (for example taking a medication daily), or they can be more complex (including having surgery or taking a radioactive iodine tablet). Thyroid treatments are very successful, and if you think you have a thyroid abnormality, be sure to discuss your concerns with your doctor.

Not using energy correctly is one main cause of fatigue. Throughout the previous chapters of this book, we've discussed oxygen and glucose as the main fuels our bodies use as energy, and I've explained that there are waste products produced as a result of our bodies' using up the oxygen and glucose. One of the primary waste products produced is carbon dioxide, and we've discussed how carbon dioxide is removed through the lungs. Besides carbon dioxide, there are many other waste products our bodies produce, and in the next several sections we'll discuss how these are removed and what happens if they aren't removed efficiently.

In general, any chemical that enters the body will eventually be removed from it. We remove waste products primarily in three ways. We've already discussed removing gases through the lungs as we **exhale** (breathe out). Another site at which waste is filtered out of the blood and disposed of is the liver, and the third pathway is through the kidneys. Our **livers** continuously filter all the blood that circulates through the body. Most chemicals that shouldn't be in the blood are taken aside as they pass through the liver and are broken down (also called **metabolized**) by the liver. As the chemicals are metabolized, byproducts are formed. Sometimes these byproducts are excreted into the intestines mixed with **bile** (a green liquid produced by the liver that not only excretes waste into the intestines but also helps digest fat that is passing through the intestines), and sometimes the waste products are passed on to the kidneys for elimination. If our livers don't function correctly (either they don't filter the chemicals well enough or they aren't able to metabolize the chemicals into byproducts that can easily be excreted), the harmful chemicals can build up. Depending on which chemicals accumulate, their buildup can cause a variety of symptoms. These symptoms can range from nausea to weight loss to fluid retention to changes in skin color (**jaundice** is the condition that results from extra **bilirubin**, which is a chemical that is put out in bile when the liver is functioning normally, remaining in the body, and as the bilirubin levels get higher, it causes the whites of the eyes and the skin to develop a yellow color), but the most common side effect of liver dysfunction is a change in mental alertness that's often described as fatigue.

Abnormal liver function can occur for a variety of reasons. The most common cause of liver failure is drinking excessive amounts of alcohol. Alcohol is among the chemicals the liver digests, but the liver can only digest so much of it at a time. If too much alcohol is in the blood, the excess alcohol that is not digested by the liver remains in the blood stream and is toxic to many parts of the body, including the liver cells themselves. The more alcohol a person drinks (either at one time or more commonly over a period of time), the more liver cells are injured and even killed. Besides alcohol consumption, there are infections (like hepatitis A, hepatitis B, and hepatitis C—we'll discuss these in more detail later) that can damage our livers; there are genetic reasons our livers can begin to malfunction; and on occasion, some medications we take can damage our livers. As liver cells are killed, they are replaced with scar tissue. Scarring of the liver is called **cirrhosis**. Cirrhosis causes a variety of different symptoms including jaundice, fluid accumulation in the belly (called **ascites**), nausea, drowsiness, and eventually death. Fortunately, our livers have extra liver cells, so they can lose a certain number of the cells yet retain normal overall liver function. However, once a critical number of liver cells is killed, the liver function will begin to decline. Unfortunately, we do not have a way to grow new liver cells, so once enough liver cells die, there is no way to get normal liver function back (aside from placing a new liver into the body through a liver transplant operation). Because liver damage is permanent and because the liver performs such a critical role, identifying and preventing liver damage before it reaches the final stages is the only way to ensure our livers continue to function adequately throughout our lives. Liver function is measured through blood tests that your doctor can order. Some tests measure irritation and damage to the liver, and some tests measure the actual performance of the liver. If you suspect your liver is not functioning normally, working with your doctor and reviewing the appropriate blood tests is the only way to determine how healthy your liver is. If your liver function is beginning to decline, identifying the cause of the liver injury and preventing further injury is the best plan of action.

The body's final area for removal of waste products is the kidneys. The **kidneys** are the body parts that create urine. Each of us has two kidneys, and our kidneys are located in our backs, under our rib cages. Just like our livers, our kidneys filter all of the blood that flows through our bodies, and they are excellent filters. Through a very complex process, they are able to get rid of most of the waste products that enter them, passing the waste products into the urine. As long as the waste products continue to flow into the urine, we do not experience any difficulties; however, if the kidneys are unable to pass all the toxins into the urine, these chemicals can build up which can lead to a variety of symptoms including fatigue. Just like with our livers, our kidneys have extra filtering capacity which means we can retain normal overall kidney function even if large numbers of kidney cells are damaged or destroyed. Also, just like our livers, once a kidney cell has been killed, we are not able create a new cell to replace it, and if enough kidney cells are damaged, overall kidney function will become inadequate. In this situation, doctors have two options to replace the lost kidney function. We can perform a kidney transplant, or we can perform **dialysis**. There are not enough kidneys available for transplant, so dialysis is the most common way we treat kidney failure. Dialysis involves passing a person's blood through a machine that filters out all the waste products. A dialysis treatment typically takes several hours, and dialysis needs to be performed several times each week in order to remove adequate amounts of waste products. While dialysis is a life-saving therapy for many people, it is neither a comfortable nor an ideal way to live, so preventing kidney failure is our goal.

Kidney damage is most commonly caused by inadequately-controlled high blood pressure or diabetes. Unfortunately, most people "feel" fine while the kidneys are being damaged by these diseases until the damage has been done and it's too late. This is

71

among the many reasons it's critically important to identify hypertension and diabetes as soon as they develop and to control them as strictly as possible once they are diagnosed. The best way to manage both hypertension and diabetes is by working very closely with your doctor. Ultimately, most people have to take medications for these diseases. Unfortunately, all medications have potential side effects, so when a person starts taking a medication to treat a disease, he may start to notice those side effects. He may soon realize that he "feels" better when he doesn't take the medication. This sometimes causes him to stop taking the medication. Before stopping any medication, it's important to weigh the benefits each medicine provides against its side effects. If the benefits are greater, it makes sense to keep taking the medication; if not, it makes sense to stop taking it. In the case of medications that are used to treat hypertension and diabetes, the degree of side effects experienced needs to be weighed against living life with permanent kidney injury, a heart attack, or a stroke. If the side effects are severe enough, discuss with your doctor changing your medications rather than simply not taking them. From a doctor's perspective, my goal is to prevent the long-term complications associated with inadequately-controlled diabetes and hypertension, so I want to do everything I can to help my patients keep these diseases under tight control in order to prevent heart attacks, strokes, and kidney failure. I encourage my patients to keep taking their medications if possible. If one medication causes significant side effects, I work very hard with my patients to find another medication that will hopefully provide the same benefits with fewer side effects. Ultimately, I understand that some people don't like taking their medications. For these folks, I do my best to help them understand the risks associated with not treating their diseases, and I offer them the option of not taking the medications as long as they're are willing to accept the risk of these very serious potential complications.

Besides managing blood pressure and blood glucose levels, doctors also want to identify any damage that might be occurring as early as possible so we can prevent more serious complications later. Understanding that hypertension and diabetes can damage several body parts, including the kidneys, doctors routinely monitor multiple aspects of body function. If we start to notice signs of injury, we may try to lower the blood pressure or blood sugar further, even if the readings obtained by the patient and/or the doctor have been "normal" up until that point. Again, the most important aspect of blood pressure and blood sugar control is the prevention of damage to the various body parts caused by these diseases. For this reason, understanding these potential complications is very important for patients so they can better work with their doctors.

For many folks, an increase in cardiovascular exercise, accompanied by weight loss, can reduce the amount of medication needed to adequately control blood pressure and blood sugar. In order to achieve the maximal benefit, exercise should elevate a person's heart rate and get her to the point that she needs to breathe more deeply and more rapidly than normal in order to keep doing the exercise. This type of **cardiovascular exercise** has been shown to have the greatest impact on blood pressure and blood sugar, and doing this exercise for at least 20 minutes each day provides the best result. I tell my patients that, if they can exercise and still carry on a normal conversation with a friend, this intensity of exercise is not providing the maximal benefit (again, they should be breathing harder and faster than normal which makes it difficult to talk normally). Patients often explain to me that they sweat a lot when they work out and that they assume that heavy sweating means they are getting a good workout. I then explain that, while sweating is the body's response to being hot, it is not necessarily a measurement of how much exercise has been performed. For this reason, I again encourage my patients to pay closer attention to their breathing rather than their sweating. Another good way to ensure you are getting an adequate level of exercise during your workout is to use a heart rate monitor. These devices can range from units that clip onto a finger, attach to a wrist, or are integrated into a piece of workout machinery. Heart rate monitors keep track of your pulse as you exercise, and the goal

73

when using a heart rate monitor is to keep your heart rate within a certain range for at least 20 minutes. The typical recommended range is between 50% and 65% of your maximum predicted heart rate, and your maximum predicted heart rate is often calculated by taking 220 and subtracting your age. For example, if you're 40 years old, your maximum predicted heart rate would be 220-40=180, and 50-65% of 180 would be 90-117 beats per minute (BPM). By this formula, your goal would be to exercise intensely enough to keep your heart rate between 90 and 117 BPM for at least 20 minutes in a row. If you're 70 years old, your maximum predicted heart rate would be 220-70=150, and 50-65% of 150 would be 75-97 BPM. This would be your target heart rate during your cardiovascular exercise routine. These target heart rates are very rough calculations, and when first starting an exercise program, be sure to use caution as you approach these targets. If you ever have any concern about the safety of your calculated target heart rate, or if you would like a more personalized target heart rate calculated for you, talk to your doctor or a personal trainer about your specific medical conditions and your level of fitness, and ask them for help in establishing a target heart rate specifically for you. Understanding that each of my patients is at a different level of physical fitness, I encourage them to start off with as much exercise as they can and to increase that level of exercise each week until they achieve at least 20 minutes of cardiovascular exercise each day. Walking to and from the mailbox is better than sitting on the couch, and increasing the length of the walk to a block, then a mile, then transitioning to a slow jog can make all the difference. We also see significant benefits with weight loss, and these benefits are seen when a person loses at least 5% of her current body weight, with the most significant benefits seen when a person reduces her weight to within a normal body mass index (BMI) (we'll discuss weight loss in more detail later). Exercise and weight loss can always be used as part of the management plan for diabetes and hypertension, and the more exercise and weight loss achieved, the less medicine will likely be needed to control these diseases. Unfortunately, it can take time to work up to a full cardiovascular exercise program, and weight loss can be a very slow process. To make matters worse, a delay in controlling diabetes and hypertension can lead to long-term complications. For this reason, I typically recommend that my patients start taking medications as soon as these diseases are diagnosed in an effort to get them under control as quickly as possible. As my patients get into a regular exercise program and begin to lose weight, we wean off the medications. The end result is that we can achieve good control of diabetes and hypertension using the least amount of medicine necessary. Whichever method we use to accomplish the goal of controlling a person's diabetes and hypertension, the real key is to identify these diseases early and manage them aggressively in an attempt to prevent long-term damage to the most sensitive and critical parts of the body.

Besides filtering out the unwanted chemicals, the kidneys actively control the levels of "wanted" substances. Calcium, sodium, and potassium are among the chemicals required by our bodies to perform their daily tasks. They are used by every cell, but they are especially important to the functioning of our nerves. Nerves are essentially like wires in our bodies, and their main function is to pass electricity from one part of the body to another. At numerous sites throughout our bodies, there are connections between two nerves or between a nerve and another body part. These connections are called **synapses** (synapses are very much like the electrical junction boxes in our houses). At these synapses, there are small spaces, and the nerve endings use electrolytes (and other chemicals at times) to pass messages across these spaces. Having normal amounts of these electrolytes in the synapses is critical for proper transmission of signals along the lengths of the nerves. If these electrolytes are not present in proper concentrations, the signals will not travel down the nerves correctly, causing the associated body parts to malfunction. Since the brain is a large collection of nerves and synapses, altered levels of calcium, sodium, and potassium can distort the transmission of signals within the brain, causing the person to be drowsy and less responsive than normal. This is often experienced as fatigue. In order to maintain normal brain function, normal levels of calcium, sodium, and potassium are critical. For most people, the kidneys are very capable of maintaining the correct levels of these electrolytes in our bodies. Similar to our earlier discussion regarding the kidneys' ability to maintain normal total body water levels, our kidneys are able to maintain normal levels of sodium, potassium, and calcium under most circumstances. For people with normal kidneys, we can take in just about as much sodium, potassium, and calcium as we want, and our kidneys are able to keep what we need and get rid of the excess. This means that monitoring and controlling dietary sodium, potassium, and calcium intake is probably not necessary for most people with normal kidney function. However, for some people (especially those people with hypertension , diabetes, and other diseases that can influence kidney function, as well as for those people who are on medications that affect kidney function), the amount of sodium, potassium, and calcium taken into the body needs to be monitored and controlled. While it's possible for us to measure and track the amounts of these electrolytes we are consuming in our diets, in order to determine how effectively our kidneys are adjusting the levels of these chemicals in our blood (which is what's important for our nerve function), we perform blood tests. Working with your doctor is the best way to figure out where you stand currently and how you may need to alter your electrolyte intake.

Besides affecting nerve function, electrolytes have profound effects on muscle function as well. Calcium is the main electrolyte responsible for causing a muscle to contract then relax. Every time you "tell" a muscle to move, the electrical signal passes from your brain, through a nerve, to the muscle. The muscle cells then release a burst of calcium that makes the muscle squeeze or "contract." When you no longer want the muscle to contract, your brain sends another signal through a nerve to the muscle, and the muscle moves the calcium back into storage, allowing the muscle to relax. With abnormal calcium levels (either too high or too low) the muscles may not contract or relax when they are supposed to, and when they do contract, the contractions may not be as forceful as they should be. Incomplete or inadequate muscle contraction is typically referred to as weakness, and as discussed in chapter 1, this is commonly confused with fatigue. Since calcium is involved in muscle function as well as in nerve function (including brain function), incorrect calcium levels can cause both weakness and fatigue, so ensuring we have adequate calcium levels in our blood is very important. For this reason, when there is concern about the possibility of either abnormal muscle function or abnormal nerve function, one of the key electrolytes we check is calcium.

As we just reviewed, the kidneys are the primary organs responsible for controlling blood calcium levels. There are two ways in which they do this: they can hold onto calcium themselves, and they can stimulate the intestines to absorb extra calcium. If the kidneys sense that the level of calcium in the blood is too low, they can prevent calcium from being excreted into the urine. If the level is too high, they can excrete extra calcium into the urine. Excretion and retention of calcium from the kidneys is one method they use to maintain normal blood calcium levels. The other method involves affecting how much calcium the intestines absorb. The kidneys exert their effect on the intestines with vitamin D. (**Vitamin D** is a chemical that is present in some foods we eat and is also produced by our skin when our skin is exposed to sunlight.) Vitamin D starts off in an "inactive" form and is "activated" by the kidneys. It's the active form of vitamin D that stimulates the intestines to absorb more calcium. When the kidneys sense that the blood calcium levels are too low, they create more activated vitamin D. When there's enough calcium in the blood, they reduce the production of this active form of vitamin D. With higher levels of activated vitamin D in the blood, the intestines respond by absorbing more calcium (if there's extra calcium available in the intestines to be absorbed). With lower levels of activated vitamin D in the blood, the intestines will absorb less calcium, even if it is available in the intestines. The balance among blood calcium levels, inactive vitamin D levels, active vitamin D levels, and levels of calcium in the intestines is very delicate. Unfortunately, it's not uncommon for these chemicals to shift out of balance.

However, we have an emergency backup system that prevents the blood calcium levels from dropping too low, even when our kidneys and intestines aren't able to keep up with our bodies' demands for calcium. The emergency backup is the calcium that we have in our bones. Unlike any other electrolyte, calcium is stored in large surplus quantities. In emergency situations, when our blood calcium levels are getting low and there isn't enough calcium in our intestines or enough activated vitamin D being produced by our kidneys, our bodies can raise the blood calcium levels by pulling extra calcium from the bones. There are two hormones that control this movement of calcium into and out of the bones. **Calcitonin** is the hormone the body releases when it senses that the blood calcium levels are getting too high. Calcitonin is produced by the **thyroid gland** (a small gland located in the front of the neck), and it causes extra calcium to move from the blood into the bones. **Parathyroid hormone**, on the other hand, is released when the blood calcium levels are getting too low. Parathyroid hormone is produced by the **parathyroid glands** (a collection of four small glands located behind the thyroid gland in the front of the neck), and it causes extra calcium to be released from the bones into the blood. In time, as more and more calcium leaves the bones, **osteoporosis** (a situation in which an abnormally low amount of calcium is present in the bones, making them weak and susceptible to breaking) can develop. Since osteoporosis can lead to hip and spinal fractures, preventing osteoporosis has become a very important goal for doctors. We'll discuss osteoporosis in more detail later in the book, but for now, be aware that keeping blood calcium levels normal through adequate calcium and vitamin D intake through our diets is important for our body's energy level and for our muscle strength as well as for maintenance of good bone health. While tracking dietary intake of calcium is possible for most folks, monitoring and adjusting blood calcium levels requires blood tests that need to be ordered and interpreted by your doctor. If you have any concerns about your bone health or about your blood calcium levels, be sure to discuss your concerns with your doctor so she can determine the best steps to take to adequately evaluate and treat your concerns.

We've discussed the fact that the brain is a large collection of nerves and synapses and that, within the synapses of our brains, there's a complex mixture of chemicals used to pass along information. The mechanism used to pass information from place to place within the brain is extraordinarily complex, utilizing different chemicals at various locations in variable amounts to send the correct information to the correct locations. The array of chemicals and concentrations and locations is so complex, in fact, that we do not fully understand the details of how it all works; however, our knowledge is advancing and has advanced dramatically in the past two decades. One area where this is most evident is in our understanding of mood changes such as anxiety and depression. Today, our best understanding of the main cause of depression and anxiety is a chemical imbalance within our brains. The chemical that most of our research has focused on to this point has been **serotonin** (one of the many chemicals that pass between the synapses of our brains). Although it appears that there are several other chemicals involved in the process as well (including **epinephrine**, **norepinephrine**, and **dopamine**), serotonin appears to be the most influential on mood. Serotonin is involved in the passing of information from the parts of our brains that record the facts of an event to the parts of our brains that experience the emotions associated with an event. For example, if we witness an automobile accident, the fact-oriented parts of our brains may remember seeing one car crash into the other, but the emotion-oriented parts may remember the fright and sadness we experienced due to the accident. It's serotonin that allows these two parts of our brains to share information, and it's this sharing of information that allows us to have a normal emotional response to various events. The passage of information between the two parts of the brain requires a certain quantity of serotonin, and different events require different quantities of serotonin for the information to pass correctly. Since different people have different levels of serotonin within their brains, some people have no difficulty with the factual and the emotional parts of their brains communicating while others are not able to perform this type of communication effectively. If the level of serotonin within a person's brain isn't sufficient to allow him to process the information of an event, or if multiple events occur all at once and the processing of this combination of events requires more serotonin than he has available at that time, he will experience a mood change, typically either depression or anxiety. As it turns out, mood changes are often accompanied by changes in energy levels which means that people who suffer from depression often suffer from fatigue as well. This connection between depression and fatigue appears to be due to the way the brain processes and passes on the perception of how much energy a person has, and again, this is related to the quantity of serotonin available in the brain. As we look for ways to treat anxiety and depression, counseling and relaxation are often helpful. Counseling and relaxation techniques appear to help reduce the amount of serotonin needed to process an event or a combination of events, but these treatment techniques don't appear to affect the brain's serotonin levels themselves. For this reason, these methods may help some people deal with stressful situations while other people may require medications to help with their mood changes. Since the brain appears to only make a certain amount of serotonin, giving the patient supplemental serotonin in the form of a medication would seem to be the best way to help people who are experiencing depression and anxiety. Unfortunately, increasing the amount of serotonin within the brain is not easy because there is a filter surrounding the brain that only allows certain chemicals that are floating around in the blood to enter. This filter is called the **blood-brain barrier (BBB)**. Unfortunately, serotonin is not able to pass through the BBB, so adding serotonin to the blood (which is what we do when we use serotonin-containing medications), does not increase the levels of serotonin in the brain where they are needed. Since doctors did not have a way to add serotonin directly to the brain, we developed medications that made the serotonin already in the brain work more effectively. These medications are called **selective serotonin reuptake inhibitors (SSRIs)**, and they work by making the serotonin that is in the synapses stay in those synapses longer than normal. This means that the synapses exposed to SSRIs will have a stronger response than we would normally see with a given amount of serotonin release.   There are many commercially-produced SSRIs on the market (many of these medications also affect the functional levels of epinephrine, norepinephrine, and/or dopamine within the brain as well), and there are numerous new SSRIs being released each year. Besides the pharmaceutical-grade SSRIs, it appears that **St. John's wort** is an herbal form of a very mild SSRI.   The SSRIs have been one of the most successful groups of medications that have been discovered in the past 20 years, and improvements continue to appear. These medications are very effective for treating anxiety and depression, and they have limited side effects. Since there are so many SSRIs available and since each one is slightly different, it can take time to find the optimal medication and dosage for each patient. Working very closely with your physician is the best way to find the best SSRI for you and to adjust the dosage so it provides you with the best control of your symptoms with the fewest side effects.

Serotonin's effects on the brain and its exact mechanism of action are not completely understood. Within our bodies, there are numerous other systems and chemical mixtures about which we have a similarly incomplete understanding. Our immune systems are an example. They are built to protect us from infection and help us heal from injury using a complex combination of protective immune cells that release a mixture of chemicals to do the job. We know that certain chemicals are involved in the response our bodies generate in order to fight off the things they see as being potential invaders, but what all these chemicals are and exactly how they all interact isn't quite clear. Some of them attract more immune cells into the area being attacked which means that once an immune response is started, a chain reaction of immune activity is initiated. Sometimes, we can see and feel this chain reaction as it develops. The area being defended typically becomes red and swollen and warm and tender. These four symptoms relate to enhanced immune activity. Another term we use for this enhanced immune activity is **inflammation**, and the chemicals that are released as part of this inflammatory response are called **inflammatory mediators**. Instead of being localized to a specific area, sometimes the perceived threat is present throughout the whole body. Subsequently, these inflammatory mediators are released and circulate everywhere. This general state of inflammation can cause us to experience fatigue if it is ongoing. Please keep in mind that there are numerous inflammatory mediators and that I will discuss just a few of the best understood. There are probably a number of inflammatory mediators that have not yet been discovered, and among those that have been discovered, the role each plays in the inflammatory process is not fully understood. This limited understanding also applies to the ones I will mention. Ongoing research on the topic of chronic inflammation, the chemicals involved, and the ways to manipulate these chemicals is very exciting and is likely to provide us with cures to many of the diseases that afflict us today.

When our bodies are exposed to something they don't like, they unleash a cascade of chemicals in order to defeat and destroy the offenders. Some of the names of these immune mediators are **immunoglobulins, cytokines, leukotrienes, compliment, chemotactic factors, and prostaglandins**. These chemicals are released, one after the other, as our bodies prepare their armies for battle. To understand and remember the names of all these chemicals isn't important, but to understand that there is a chain reaction that occurs once our immune systems are stimulated is important. This response is designed to destroy the offender, but, unfortunately, there is often collateral damage associated with the destruction of the foreign item. This means that normal, healthy cells in the area of the invasion are often damaged along with the invading item itself. This is important to remember because prolonged exposure to these inflammatory mediators can cause excessive wear and tear on our bodies. Typically, our bodies are able to grow new cells and recover from the injury, but with a prolonged exposure to these chemicals, the body parts under attack can be permanently injured. As with most other systems in our bodies, there are checks and balances within the immune system. As local inflammation increases, the brain (unconsciously) tries to keep the inflammation from getting out of control and at the same time alert the rest of the body to get ready for a possible spread of the invasion. The brain, through what we call the **stress response**, sends a signal to the **adrenal glands** (small clusters of cells that sit on top of the kidneys and produce a variety of different hormones) to release steroids that are the messengers used to modify the body's immune response. These steroids aren't the same kind that body builders take in order to grow their muscles. These steroids are called **glucocorticoids** (one well-known glucocorticoid is called **cortisol**). The exact complex sequence of effects glucocorticoids have on all parts of the immune system aren't fully understood, but one of their effects is to slow the production and release of the chemicals of inflammation. Unfortunately, these steroids not only affect the immune system, but they also affect numerous other parts of the body as well. They can cause us to retain fluid leading to swelling in our legs and even in our arms and faces. They can alter our metabolism causing our bodies to begin to break down muscle cells instead of fat cells when we need more energy. Glucocorticoids can cause our bones, hair, skin, and nails to begin to break down and become fragile and thin. Glucocorticoids can cause our bodies to use glucose inefficiently which can cause our blood sugars to go up. Under the influence of glucocorticoids, our brains may not process information properly. Many people become **manic** (have an uncontrollable amount of energy that can keep them from sleeping at night and can cause them to make decisions and take actions they wouldn't normally), and some people even become psychotic and experience **hallucinations** (seeing or hearing things that aren't really there) and **delusions** (having strong beliefs that something is true even when given facts proving that it is not true). These aberrations can occur to varying degrees in different people, but the constant wear and tear put on our bodies when glucocorticoid levels are chronically elevated almost always eventually produce some degree of harmful effects.

One of the side effects of chronic inflammation is chronic fatigue, and unfortunately, there are many sources of fatigue-causing chronic inflammation. Some of these sources are common, and some are rare. Among the most common are allergic reactions to environmental chemicals. Allergies can develop to a wide array of substances (called **allergens**) present in our environments, and they can lead to a variety of different symptoms. The most common irritating chemicals are cigarette smoke, dust and dust mites, pollen, pets (especially ones with fur or feathers), and molds and mildews. The immune systems of people with allergies overreact to these chemicals, and the inflammatory cascade begins. Allergies can present with inflammation of the lungs (called **asthma**), inflammation of the skin (often called **eczema**), or inflammation of the nose (called **rhinitis**). If the allergen is present in high-enough concentrations for long enough, elevated levels of inflammatory mediators and glucocorticoids may be released, giving us chronic fatigue. Treatment of allergic conditions involves eliminating as many allergens as possible. For some folks, this means they cannot have certain pets. For others, it may involve using special HEPA filters on vacuums and on furnaces, and for others, it may involve more radical environmental modifications like removing carpeting and putting plastic covers on pillows and mattresses. There are medications commonly used to treat these allergic diseases, and discussing the correct mixture of environmental modification and medication with your doctor is important when trying to control the fatigue associated with chronic allergic conditions.

Another circumstance in which our bodies experience similarly elevated levels of inflammation and, therefore, fatigue, is when we have chronic infections. Our immune systems are designed to fight infections, and they do so by releasing their cascades of inflammatory mediators. If we are constantly fighting infections, there will be consistently increased levels of inflammatory mediators circulating, and this can make us feel fatigued. Among the most common causes of chronic infections are the **hepatitis B and hepatitis C** viruses. The term "**hepatitis**" means inflammation of the liver. The liver can be inflamed (or irritated) by a variety of different substances with the most common being alcohol and infection. As researchers discovered different viruses that were causing infections of the liver, they named the viruses with progressive letters. The first virus was, therefore, called hepatitis A. The second was hepatitis B. The third was hepatitis C. The forth was hepatitis D and so on. At this point, scientists are up to hepatitis G. You'll never run into most of these because they are rare causes of significant infections in humans, but some very common. **Hepatitis A** is typically spread through food. A person who has an infection with hepatitis A passes the virus through his intestines. If an infected person has a bowel movement and does not wash his hands well enough, the virus can remain on his hands. If he then touches food, the virus can pass onto the food. If the food is one that is typically eaten raw (like a fruit or a vegetable) and if the food isn't washed adequately, the live virus can be eaten by someone else who can then develop a new infection. An infection with the hepatitis A virus can make a person sick, but the infection typically goes away fairly quickly without any long-term complications. Interestingly, as much as 75% of all adults in the United States show evidence of having had hepatitis A infection at some point in their lives, and most didn't have any symptoms or thought the symptoms were caused by "the flu". Good hand washing and washing of fresh fruits and vegetables is the primary way to prevent the spread of hepatitis A. Since a small number of people can get very sick if they get an infection with hepatitis A, there is now a vaccine used to prevent it. The vaccine is now routinely given to children, and it's recommended for adults who will be traveling to countries where hygiene and food preparation standards might be low. If you are planning a trip to an area where you feel there's an increased risk of catching hepatitis A, discuss your trip with your doctor, and consider getting the hepatitis A vaccine if you haven't already had it. If you are considering a trip to an area where there's an increased risk of catching other infections, visiting a **travel medicine doctor** at a **travel medicine clinic** might be the best way to ensure you are maximally protected for your trip. The other two important forms of hepatitis are **hepatitis B** and **hepatitis C**. These viruses are spread through sexual contact, through using needles that have infected blood on them (including needles used to inject drugs or needles used to apply tattoos), and through receiving blood transfusions. These viruses are much more dangerous than the hepatitis A virus because hepatitis B and C can cause chronic infections meaning the viruses may live in a person's body for the rest of his life. A person with a chronic hepatitis infection may feel fine, or he may feel ill. A person with a chronic hepatitis infection can spread the virus to other people, and since some people with chronic hepatitis infections feel fine, the infected person can spread the virus to other people without knowing he is spreading the infection (or put another way, people can catch the virus without knowing they are being exposed and infected). Eventually, most people who have chronic hepatitis have symptoms. Along with the symptoms of liver infection (pain, nausea, fatigue, jaundice), these viruses cause physical damage to the liver. This damage leads to scarring, and when enough scar tissue has formed within the liver, we call this **cirrhosis of the liver**. The damage can also cause the liver cells to mutate, leading to the development of cancer. In the body's attempt to fight the infection, inflammatory mediators are released. If the infection persists, these substances can be present indefinitely, leading to the numerous complications of chronic inflammation, including fatigue. Furthermore, as the infection spreads, it damages more and more liver cells. In time, there may be so few liver cells alive and functioning that the person may suffer **liver failure,** and the liver will be unable to keep up with its filtering job. With liver failure, our body's waste products begin to build up, and as the waste products accumulate and the inflammatory mediators circulate, we feel more and more fatigued. When a person gets to this stage of liver infection, we have no treatment for the disease aside from liver transplant. Currently, preventing the spread of hepatitis B and C is based on avoiding unprotected sexual contact and exposure to contaminated needles or contaminated blood products. Avoiding exposure to the hepatitis viruses is the best option, but we are always looking for other ways to prevent the spread of these infections. Currently, there is a very effective vaccination against the hepatitis B virus, and many people were immunized against hepatitis B as children. The vaccine protects most people from becoming infected during exposure to the virus, and there are very few side effects from the vaccine. Chronic hepatitis B infection is a miserable disease, so the vaccine is very worthwhile in order to protect people in the event that they would unknowingly be exposed to the virus. Unfortunately, we do not yet have a vaccine against hepatitis C, so avoiding potential exposure is the only way we have to prevent the spread of the disease. When these chronic infections were first discovered, doctors thought we could "tell" who had an infection and who didn't, based on what people looked like. Unfortunately, we quickly learned that people who "appeared" to be completely healthy could have a chronic infection. Since people with chronic infections may look completely healthy and since we can't tell who might be infected, we have to be very cautious so we don't catch an infection unexpectedly. For this reason, universal precautions were developed. In a healthcare setting, universal precautions are used to protect healthcare workers from an accidental exposure to an unexpected infection. **Universal precautions** involve treating everyone as if they might have an infection (the "universal" part means we treat everyone the same). This means that, for every patient we see, we use the same protective measures we would use on a person we knew had a chronic infection. We do this simply because there is no way to know for sure who has an infection and who does not. Hepatitis B and C are chronic, progressive infections. There are medications that are used to control hepatitis C infections, but they are expensive and have extensive side effects. There are no good treatments for hepatitis B infections unless you treat the infection immediately after exposure. For these reasons, my recommendation is to always protect yourself against infection, and if you think you may have been exposed to an infection, seek medical evaluation and treatment immediately.

Besides the various hepatitis viruses, there are other viruses and bacteria that can cause chronic infections as well. **Lyme disease** is an infection spread by bacteria-carrying deer ticks. (Incidentally, deer ticks are much smaller than their cousins the wood ticks. Deer ticks are roughly the size of the head of a pin, so it is very easy, and even very common, to not know you've been bitten by a deer tick.) The bacteria that cause the infection are called **Borrelia burgdorferi**. These bacteria live inside the deer tick and enter our bodies when the deer tick bites us. Typically, but not always, infection with Borrelia burgdorferi starts off with a local rash that looks something like a bulls eye. In time, the bacteria can infect joints and even the brain, and the damage done to these parts of the body can be permanent. If these bacteria go untreated for an extended period of time, significant complications, one of which is chronic fatigue, are possible. For this reason, treating a suspected case of Lyme disease with antibiotics (which are very effective against Borrelia burgdorferi) early in the course of the disease is the goal. Lyme disease is present only in select areas of the United States, so in most of our country, there is limited risk of infection; however, the long-term complications of an untreated infection are so significant that any time you think you've been bitten by a deer tick and you then develop any unusual symptoms, whether it's a typical rash or joint pain and swelling or unexplained fevers or changes in your mental abilities, it would be in your best interest to be seen by your doctor to determine the likelihood of your having Lyme disease. Lyme disease is treated with antibiotics, and early treatment prevents the long-term, potentially devastating, complications of an untreated infection.

Mononucleosis or "**mono**" is another disease caused by a chronic infection. Mononucleosis is caused by the **Epstein-Barr virus** (or **EBV**), and for some reason, EBV has the ability to evade our immune systems for prolonged periods of time. This infection, commonly known as "the kissing disease," is spread primarily through saliva (therefore the nickname). It can make a person feel fatigued for months, and it can cause dramatically enlarged lymph nodes. (**Lymph nodes** are clusters of immune cells located in all parts of the body—most prominently in the groin, in the armpits, and in the neck—that filter the blood and the **lymph** (which is fluid that leaks out of the blood vessels and typically carries a variety of different chemicals including immune cells). The primary goal of this filtration process is to remove infections.) The tonsils and the spleen are two other blood and lymph filtering organs. Whenever a lymph node (or the tonsils or the spleen) removes an infection from the blood or lymph, the immune response within that structure is increased, and the structure increases in size. So a lymph node (or tonsil or spleen) that is actively removing an infection will typically be large and painful. In severe cases of mononucleosis, tonsils can swell to the point that they fill up the back of a person's throat and interfere with breathing. In these situations, medications, and sometimes even hospitalization, are needed to adequately treat mononucleosis. Also, with severe mononucleosis infections, the spleen can swell to several times its normal size. Like an overfilled water balloon, a swollen spleen is fragile, and the risk of the spleen breaking becomes a significant concern. Being able to tell that your spleen is enlarged is very difficult for most people who haven't been trained in this physical exam skill, so avoiding injury to the stomach is the key to preventing a potentially life-threatening rupture of the spleen when you have mononucleosis. In most cases, mononucleosis acts like any other viral illness—a person feels sick for a few days to a week and then recovers without any problems. The most important things to do to help yourself recover quickly in these cases are to make sure you increase your rest and stay well-hydrated. Staying well-hydrated involves taking in as much liquid as you can, no matter what form the liquid comes in (soup, water, milk, ice cream, Jell-O, Popsicles and any other form of liquid are all good options). As with other viruses, preventing the spread of the infection is also important, so good hand washing and avoiding sharing saliva (through kissing or sharing utensils and cups) are good general practices. In the atypical cases of mononucleosis (situations where the sick feeling or extreme fatigue lasts for several weeks or when the tonsils are significantly swollen), working with your doctor to undergo laboratory testing to verify that mononucleosis is the cause and discussing more advanced treatment options is the safest and most effective way to treat your symptoms.

Tuberculosis has nearly been forgotten but is still active in our communities. **Tuberculosis** is an infection caused by **Mycobacterium tuberculosis**. It most commonly infects the lungs, although nearly any organ can become infected with these bacteria. Unfortunately, the symptoms are frequently so mild that a person can be infected and not be aware of it. This allows the person to unknowingly spreading the disease. Tuberculosis is most common in people from foreign countries (those in which control measures have been less successful), people who are homeless, people who live in crowded living conditions such as homeless shelters or jails, and those with abnormal immune systems caused by cancer or other chronic infections. Tuberculosis is typically spread from one person to another through infected droplets of mucous that fly through the air when the infected person coughs. A common symptom of tuberculosis is a persistent cough, often bringing up blood with mucous. Severe sweating, which is worst at night while sleeping, is typical as well. Fatigue can often be among the symptoms of tuberculosis. Screening for tuberculosis is performed with a needle prick on the arm (this test is called a **PPD** which stands for **purified protein derivative**). This test only shows whether or not your immune system recognizes the tuberculosis bacteria. It does not tell you if you have a current infection with tuberculosis. For example, this test can be positive (meaning the immune system recognizes the bacteria) in someone who had an infection in the past but who is no longer infected because he was successfully treated, and it can be negative (meaning the immune system does not recognize the bacteria) in someone who currently has an infection but whose immune system is not functioning normally. If the PPD is positive, additional testing is needed to determine if the person actually has tuberculosis. This typically includes an x-ray of the chest, and possibly a CT scan of the chest, along with collecting secretions from the lungs (usually by having the person cough up as much mucous as possible first thing each morning). The tuberculosis bacteria are very difficult to kill, so special antibiotics are used for an extended period of time if an infection is identified. The bacteria also typically wrap themselves in scar tissue (which we call **granulomas**) that blocks the immune system and the antibiotics from getting to the bacteria themselves. This makes it even more difficult to kill the bacteria. Finally, the bacteria are constantly learning how to survive exposure to antibiotics (which we call **antibiotic resistance**), so we typically use more than one antibiotic when treating tuberculosis. Overall, tuberculosis has been a very difficult disease to eliminate, and current treatment typically requires a patient to take more than one antibiotic for several months in order to be sure the bacteria are fully eliminated. For these reasons, if you or anyone you know thinks she has tuberculosis, being diagnosed as early as possible, starting antibiotics as soon as possible, and continuing the antibiotics for the full, recommended duration of treatment without missing any doses are critically important to be sure the tuberculosis infection does not persist and that the fatigue caused by the tuberculosis infection resolves.

Another common infection that can cause chronic fatigue is HIV. Although infection with the **human immunodeficiency virus (HIV)** typically starts off with symptoms that are similar to other viral infections (fever, chills, fatigue), it can be present for years with minimal symptoms. HIV spreads in a manner similar to hepatitis B and C. The virus attacks the body's immune system, making the immune system less effective. Over time, as the immune system is worn down further and further, the infected person becomes susceptible to other infections. Many of these other infections are caused by bacteria and viruses usually kept in check by a normal immune system. Once an HIV-infected person's immune system is destroyed beyond a certain point, the person is said to have **acquired immunodeficiency syndrome (AIDS)**. Over the past 30 years since it was first discovered, the diagnosis and treatment of HIV have evolved extensively. We now know that there's a period of time between when a person first comes in contact with the virus and when the virus actually establishes itself in the person's body. This means that if a person takes **antiretroviral medications** (antibiotic-like medicines that fight against certain viruses) as soon as he suspects he's been exposed to the HIV virus, the likelihood of his actually becoming infected goes down significantly. If the exposure isn't identified and antiretroviral medications aren't started, there's a period of time during which the virus is growing and taking hold of the immune system but during which we cannot detect it with our tests. We call this period of time the **window period**. One important point about the window period is that a person who has an HIV infection in the window period will test negative for HIV but can still spread the infection to other people. Once the virus has established itself, we now have improved screening tests that are rapid and accurate for detecting possible infection, and these tests can even be performed at home. If the screening test shows possible infection, we perform confirmatory blood tests. These tests have improved as well, and we now have lab tests that can help us to choose which antiretroviral medications are likely to work against specific strains of HIV. We also have very much improved antiretroviral medications that are more effective and easier to take with fewer side effects compared to some of our earlier options. A disease that, just a short time ago, was a death sentence is now manageable, but it is not yet curable. This means prevention is the key. If you are potentially exposed to the virus (remembering the principles of universal precautions which means we can't tell who is and who isn't infected just by looking at them), early consultation with your doctor becomes critically important.

Our immune systems are supposed to protect us from invasion by foreign substances trying to enter our bodies. They are supposed to be able to identify which substances are foreign and which are normal parts of our bodies. Occasionally, for some as yet unknown reason, our immune systems mistakenly see our own body parts as the enemy. When this happens, we call it an **autoimmune disease**. With autoimmune diseases, since our immune systems are activated, they will begin to stimulate the release of inflammatory mediators, igniting the inflammation cascade. Such diseases as **rheumatoid arthritis** (the immune system attacks the joints), **Crohn's disease** (the immune system attacks the intestines), and **systemic lupus erythematosus (SLE**

or just lupus) (the immune systems attacks various body parts and often starts off as a rash) represent some examples of autoimmune diseases. With these, chronic inflammation ensues, and the complications of chronic inflammation follow. Autoimmune diseases can be very difficult to diagnose because the immune responses typically fluctuate over time meaning that sometimes, the inflammation is more pronounced and sometimes less so. These diseases require a variety of different blood tests in order to make the diagnoses, and occasionally, additional testing (like a biopsy) is required. Once diagnosed, these diseases typically require medications designed to reduce our bodies' immune responses (drugs called **immunosuppressants**) to treat them, and immunosuppressants have significant potential side effects because inhibiting our immune systems reduces our bodies' protection against things like infections and cancer. Autoimmune diseases are not uncommon, but their diagnosis and treatment can be difficult. For these reasons, if you suspect you might have an autoimmune disease, talk to your doctor. Many doctors diagnose and treat autoimmune diseases, and **rheumatologists** (doctors who specialize in treating disorders of the joints and also disorders associated with inflammation) will typically have the most experience in this area.

The final cause of chronic fatigue I'd like to discuss in this chapter is **medications**. We, as physicians, interested in treating diseases in the most effective manner, prescribe medications for these disease processes. Furthermore, we as the general public, interested in taking good care of ourselves, take over-the-counter medications to relieve the symptoms that ail us. Every medication (including vitamins, minerals, and herbs) has potential side effects, and for many, one of the common side effects is fatigue. I need to make sure that I am clear about vitamins and herbals supplements at this point. These have tremendous potential for benefit; however, just because something is "natural" or "organic" does not mean that it is safe or automatically beneficial. **Botulinum toxin** is all natural and is one of the most potent nerve toxins ever discovered. **Opium** is an all-natural hallucinogen and pain medication with unparalleled addictive potential, and **kava kava** is an all-natural anxiety relieving herb that has been linked to increased risk of liver injury and even liver failure. In the process of selling a new pharmaceutical, a drug manufacturer is required to perform extensive testing and prove to the Food and Drug Administration (FDA) that the drug is safe and effective. Even when a drug looks good initially, it isn't uncommon for it to be later pulled from the market due to unexpected side effects. Additionally, every pharmaceutical manufacturer needs to prove to the FDA that the manufacturer has standardized production processes and that every pill of a particular drug contains the same amount of the active ingredient. For vitamins and herbal supplements, there are no standards that ensure a product actually does what the seller says it does, and there are no unbiased, third-party reviews performed to evaluate whether or not it causes side effects. The only time the FDA steps in is when a vitamin or an herb appears to be causing significant harm to the public. Otherwise, there is no regulation and no oversight because these products are considered food supplements, not drugs. Since there is no regulation of vitamins and herbal supplements, choosing a trusted adviser and a trusted manufacturer is critical before starting to take any of these. Before I recommend any vitamin or herbal supplement, I prefer to see that some level of scientific research has been done to verify both safety and efficacy. Also, I recommend my patients only use manufacturers who follow rigidly standardized production processes. This allows my patients to feel confident that the first capsule of **echinacea** (an herbal supplement commonly used to treat colds) they take has the same amount of active ingredient as every other capsule they take. Germany has probably done more research on vitamins and herbs than any other country, and reviewing the German research, or finding someone who will review it with you, can often be helpful in your search for good information. Be sure to do your homework before putting anything, whether it's natural, organic, or synthetic, into your body.

Almost any medication (again, including vitamins and herbal supplements) can make a person feel fatigued, and as we

94

Americans take more and more medications, there is an increasing likelihood that one of them, or a combination of them, will deplete our normal energy supplies. With that said, there are some general rules about which medicines cause more fatigue than others. We will go into this topic in much greater detail later in the book, but for now, I'll introduce some of the most common offenders that include medicines used to treat high blood pressure, those used to treat mood and other psychiatric or neurological disorders (seizures, for example), as well as ones used to treat pain. I want to be sure I emphasize that over-the-counter medications, including the vitamins, herbs, and minerals we use to treat these diseases, can cause fatigue as easily as the medications I prescribe in my office. As our population ages, more and more people will be taking increasing amounts of medication, and as the cost of prescription drugs continues to rise and as information becomes more readily available online, people will consume increasing amounts of over-the-counter products. The more chemicals we put into our bodies, the more side effects we may experience. In order to make a rational decision as to which medicines to continue and which to stop, a person needs to make sure she has a clear understanding of the benefits and the side effects of each medicine she is taking. To make this decision more difficult, the benefits may not become apparent for quite some time whereas the side effects may develop immediately. As we discussed earlier, taking blood pressure medication may prevent a heart attack several years down the road, but it may make you feel fatigued today. This means you might have a tough decision to make. If you had to choose between fatigue and a heart attack, which would you choose? These are not easy decisions, and they are made even more complex as more and more medicines are added to the equation. The only way to stay on top of your medications is to review them regularly with your doctor and your pharmacist and have a very clear understanding of the benefits and risks of each medication you take. For most diseases there are several options for medications that provide similar benefits, so if one is causing an intolerable side effect, switching to another can often provide the benefits we are looking for without the side effects. In some cases, options among the available medications are more limited, so the choice is between a more effective medicine that has more side effects and a less effective one that has fewer side effects. If you have questions about any of the medications you are taking, please ask your doctor about the likelihood of their causing your fatigue. If your medications are causing fatigue, be sure to ask if there are alternative medicines that can adequately treat your medical conditions. Make sure you understand the answers to these questions before you stop taking the medications, and as discussed above, please consider the long-term benefits of each medication before   making   your   final   decision.

Chapter 5: Causes of Fatigue— Others

To this point we've discussed causes of fatigue that we can more or less explain. For the most part, if a person is suffering from one of the previously-mentioned causes of fatigue, we can identify the cause, we have some understanding of the mechanism, and we can adopt a reasonable approach to address the problem. Unfortunately, despite our continued research and our constantly expanding knowledge, we still encounter diseases that we do not understand and that are difficult to treat. This is true with fatigue as well.

The bad news is that there are causes of fatigue that we don't understand. The good news is that many of the causes of fatigue discussed in the previous chapters weren't understood and couldn't be diagnosed in the past but can be diagnosed and are effectively treated today. Prior to our learning about congestive heart failure, for example, people would suffer with ongoing fatigue despite our treatments. This was frustrating both for the patient and the physician. Now that we understand congestive heart failure better, we have good treatments that improve the fatigue for the people who suffer with this disease. It's vital to understand that there are numerous medical diseases that we haven't yet identified which means that even if we don't have a specific diagnostic test that can definitively give a name to the specific cause of your symptoms, it doesn't mean that a real medical condition isn't causing your fatigue. Patients frequently ask me, "Am I crazy, Dr. Gariti? Is this all in my head?" I respond, "Just because WE aren't smart enough yet to know why you feel like you do, it doesn't in any way mean you're crazy. You clearly have a something going on, and someday, I will be able to tell you what causes it and how to make it better."

Unfortunately, for those people who suffer from fatigue caused by some not-yet-understood problem, we won't have specific treatment options we can offer. In these cases, we typically rely on treatments that work for other fatigue-causing medical problems and hope they'll help. Sometimes, the general treatments help, and sometimes they don't. If not, we are then faced with an ongoing search for an identifiable cause of fatigue and a trial-and-error approach to treatment. Frequently frustrated, patients and doctors alike cycle through prolonged diagnostic testing and ineffective treatments, hoping to make the symptoms go away. I will discuss some of the general strategies used to help those with undiagnosed causes of fatigue in a later chapter, but for now, let's give some names to causes of fatigue we know exist but don't really understand.

The first cause of fatigue that falls under this category is **chronic fatigue syndrome**. Chronic fatigue syndrome was first defined by the Centers for Disease Control and Prevention back in 1988 and then updated in 1994. Its definition is:

1. Have severe chronic fatigue of six months or longer duration with other known medical conditions excluded by clinical diagnosis, and

2. Concurrently have four or more of the following symptoms: substantial impairment in short-term memory or concentration, sore throat, tender lymph nodes, muscle pain, multi-joint pain without swelling or redness, headaches of a new type, pattern or severity, unrefreshing sleep, and post-exertional malaise lasting more than 24 hours.

As you can see, there is significant overlap between this definition and the symptoms we discussed earlier that are associated with some of the other causes of fatigue, and before we can make the diagnosis of chronic fatigue syndrome, we must first make sure the symptoms aren't part of another medical condition. In fact, as described in criterion number 1, we must exclude all other medical conditions prior to making the diagnosis of chronic fatigue syndrome.   Unfortunately, excluding other medical conditions can take some time and will require extensive testing, all of which must be normal in order to make this diagnosis. Waiting and wondering, patients and physicians frequently become confused and frustrated with fatigue and sometimes give up on trying to figure out what is wrong and how to make it better. Don't give up. Keep working with your doctor. Find a support group in your area to help you get through the waiting and wondering. There is significant research being done on chronic fatigue syndrome, and someday, we'll understand its cause. While you're working on the diagnosis, there are some general techniques you can use to improve your energy level, and we'll discuss these in a later chapter.

The other symptom complex that is frequently frustrating and complicated to diagnose and treat is **fibromyalgia**. The concept of fibromyalgia has been in existence for many years, although there was, and still remains, confusion about its cause. To allow doctors to diagnose and track the disease, the American College of Rheumatology developed criteria that describe fibromyalgia. These criteria include having pain on both sides (left and right) of the body, as well as having pain above and below the waist. This pain must be present for at least three months, and there must be tenderness at 11 out of 18 specific locations when those locations are pushed on. Although there is some debate about the importance of tenderness at specific sites, the 18 sites described by the American College of Rheumatology include the left and right sides of the body at the following locations: The bottom of the skull in the back of the head, near the middle of the neck in the back of the neck, the point where the neck and the shoulders meet in the back, the point where the neck and the shoulders meet in the front, just below the collar bone where the rib meets the breast bone, the outside part of the elbow, the part of the hip bone that sticks out farthest, the muscles that make up the buttocks, and the inside part of the knee. Fibromyalgia is frequently associated with severe fatigue. The relationship between this fatigue and the pain of fibromyalgia isn't clear. It's possible that fibromyalgia and fatigue interact similarly to chronic pain and fatigue in that being in constant pain is stressful which wears a person out. There's also the possibility that whatever chemical change in the body causes a person to experience fibromyalgia also directly causes the person to feel fatigued. Research is ongoing in our attempt to better understand fibromyalgia, and at this point we continue to treat fibromyalgia by using medications we use for other painful or fatigue-causing medical problems.

It's clearly possible to feel fatigued without meeting the rest of the criteria for a specific syndrome. In this case, I would again encourage you to be patient and persistent. Work through the steps necessary to ensure you don't have another, already defined, medical problem. Work with your doctor through some general treatment options I'll describe later in the book, and keep in mind that, as more and more research is done on fatigue-causing illnesses, there will be more options available to treat your fatigue.

Section II: How to Figure Out What is Causing Your Fatigue

How to Figure Out What is Causing Your Fatigue

Chapter 6: What Can You Do on Your Own?

Arriving at this point in the book, you can appreciate how many different causes of fatigue there are, and you have a basic understanding of some of the ways we go about identifying certain ones. In this section of the book, I will discuss in more detail the steps you can take at home, as well as the steps your doctors might take in an effort to answer the question of why you have the symptoms you have. These next two chapters are designed to help you identify the path that leads to an improvement in your symptoms, and the final section of the book will describe the steps you can take that will move you down that path.

As discussed earlier, the majority of people who are experiencing fatigue feel the way they do because they are not getting restful sleep on a regular basis. Because sleep alterations are so common, evaluating sleep habits is a crucial first step toward finding the cause for the majority of the cases of fatigue. The exact amount of sleep each night, as well as the reasons for not sleeping, are pieces of information that are readily available to us. All we have to do is pay attention. For most people, acquiring the details of why they are experiencing difficulties with their sleep can be a relatively simple task.   The solution is a sleep diary. A **sleep diary** consists of pieces of paper on which we record all the information about our sleep habits each night.   As we begin tracking the details of our sleep difficulties, many reasons for not sleeping quickly become obvious.   For a sleep diary to provide valuable information, it needs to track certain key events during each night's sleep.   These events need to include activities performed before going to sleep, activities surrounding falling asleep, and activities surrounding waking up.   Along with each event, we need to record the time it occurred, and we need to list the thoughts, feelings, or other influences related to each event.

The information should be recorded as soon after the event as possible (ideally while experiencing the event) which means the diary needs to be kept next to our beds and we need to write in our diaries every time an event happens, even when the event occurs in the middle of the night. Waking ourselves in the middle of the night to write information in a sleep diary will provide the most accurate information, and while we may be tempted to try to remember all the events that occurred throughout the night and then write them all down in the morning, by the time we wake up, many of the critical details of why the sleep was interrupted will be lost...our drowsy brains can only remember so much for so long. Taking a few extra moments to write things down as they are happening will ultimately provide the best information which will give us the best chance of finding the causes of any sleep disturbances. The bad news is that the process will take some effort. The good news is that we do not need to do this forever.

Let's take a look at one of my patients. We'll call her Sally. After dinner, Sally reads a book, goes to sleep, and then wakes up in the morning to go to work. If she were to simply come to my office without a sleep diary, she might describe her night's sleep by saying, "nothing much happened last night." But if she were to bring in a good sleep diary it might look like something like this:

Event	Time	Thought
Prepare for bed	10:30-11:30pm	I want to relax before bed.
Go to bed	12:00am	I really need to get some sleep. I have a busy day tomorrow. I hope I don't wake up tonight.
Sleep	1:00am	
Awake	2:30am	My spouse went to the bathroom.
Try to go back to sleep	2:35am	I really need some sleep.
Sleep	2:45am	
Awake	4:00am	I have to go to the bathroom.
Try to go back to sleep	4:15am	I hope I'm not tired tomorrow. I have a long day ahead of me.
Sleep	4:45am	
Awake	6:00am	Darn alarm! I'm still tired.

Once we see her sleep diary, it doesn't take much effort to obtain clues about Sally's sleep problems. Her sleep diary shows us that, even if she had slept the entire night without interruption, she would have only slept six hours which is probably not enough. Again, most of us require at least eight hours of sleep to be completely rested, so scheduling at least eight hours for sleep each night is a good start. As we continue to look at the sleep diary, we can also see that it took Sally approximately one hour to fall asleep. Normally, falling asleep should only take ten to twenty minutes, and when this process takes longer than normal, we call it **prolonged sleep latency**. Was there a reason Sally's onset of sleep was delayed? Was the book Sally was reading scary or exceptionally thought-provoking? Had she had a stressful day?

Was she thinking about tomorrow's busy schedule? Was it too warm or too cold in the house that night? Was there a storm outside? Every bit of detail helps us understand possible reasons why Sally's sleep was affected. Our goal with this process is to identify the causes of sleep disturbances and to control the disturbances we can control. Avoiding exciting TV shows or books before bed, performing relaxation techniques (like taking a hot shower or meditating) just before going to bed, adjusting the environment (temperature, air flow, and light in the room), and wearing ear plugs and/or a sleep mask in order to block out the environment around us are all adjustments that are easy to make yet can have profound benefits.

The next group of sleep disturbances identified in the sleep diary is bed partner-related issues—Sally's husband, Fred, wakes up in the middle of the night and wakes Sally in the process. Why is he waking up? Is he noisy when he sleeps? Does he snore or talk while sleeping? Does he toss and turn? Does he routinely steal her covers? All of these issues can wake Sally causing frequent awakenings, incomplete sleep cycles, and fatigue. Once identified, bed partner issues can be resolved. Of course, Fred could perform a sleep diary of his own in an effort to identify any sleep issues he might have, and he could discuss his problems with his doctor which could lead to resolution of both his problems and Sally's as well. If Fred continued to be restless at night, Sally could look for ways to limit Fred's impact on her sleep. Buying a motion-resistant bed or using two separate mattresses might prevent Sally from being awoken by Fred's movements at night. Having two separate sets of blankets could ensure Sally remained covered throughout the night. Wearing ear plugs and a sleeping mask would help Sally ignore Fred's nocturnal activities. As Sally reviews her sleep diary, she's looking for correctable causes of her sleep problems, and if Sally identifies that Fred is part of her repeated nocturnal awakenings, she and Fred need to work together to find ways to improve both her sleep and his.

Besides bed partner issues, a very common cause of interruption of sleep is children. Do your children come into your bedroom frequently throughout the night, waking you? Do they need drinks in the middle of the night? Do they get hot or cold? Do they hear noises that scare them? Most children love their parents, and most children want as much attention from their parents as they can get. Just like the child who calls to her mother, "Mommy, look at me!" while she rides her bike along the sidewalk, most children want to be acknowledged and praised at every opportunity. Most of the time, the same driving force causes a child to ask for a drink of water at night or leads a child to knock on your bedroom door and ask if she can sleep with you—she is seeking your attention. With very few exceptions, a child knocking at your door or coming into your bed at night is doing so primarily as a means of spending more time with you. In general, there's nothing wrong with a child's attention seeking; however, there are more and less appropriate times to give that attention to your child. Most of us would agree that, if a child called to us, asking us to look at a drawing she completed at school, we would not hesitate to look, but if she asked us to look at her drawing while we were driving through heavy traffic in a rain storm, we would insist that we wait until we got home. The child is physically and mentally capable of waiting until we get home before we look at the drawing, and no long-term harm will come to her if we wait until we are in a safe and appropriate location. Conversely, immediate harm may come to us and her if we decide to look at the drawing while driving. The same concept applies to children disturbing our sleep. If we find we are not getting enough sleep at night and at least part of our sleep disturbance is related to our children waking us at night, we have to acknowledge that children typically come to our rooms at night merely in an effort to seek attention. This is an inappropriate time for our children to seek our attention. Children need to be taught that there are appropriate times to seek attention and that there are inappropriate ones, and we, the parents, are the ones who need to teach our children this lesson. If your daughter comes to you in the middle of the night asking for a drink of water, telling her that she can get her own drink or that you will get her a drink in the morning is a reasonable response. If your son was tucked in at bedtime and now comes to your room asking to be tucked in again, telling him to go back to bed and that you won't tuck him in again tonight is a reasonable response. Teaching our children that they should not expect attention from us at inappropriate times will not cause them any long-term harm. Conversely, allowing our children to repeatedly wake us at night to fulfill these requests for attention can cause us and our children immediate and long-term harm if we are constantly sleep deprived and feel chronically fatigued.

We also need to realize that a large part of the reason children continue to come to our rooms at night is because we have trained them to do so. Our children are smart, and they learn from their experiences. They are always seeking new ways to get the things they want, and when they find a successful technique, they keep using it until it doesn't work anymore. It's not uncommon for a child who wants candy while at the grocery store to ask his parents over and over if he can have the candy. If, after the fifth request, the parents get frustrated and buy the child the candy, the child learns that the best way to get candy from his parents is to ask repeatedly. From then on, he will use his proven technique. On the other hand, if the parents never give in to his requests and instead only buy him candy when he behaves in a way they want him to behave (perhaps he only gets candy after he's helped put the groceries in the car and gotten into his car seat), he will learn that lesson as well. Now that he's learned this new way to get the candy he wants, this will be the habit he will repeat in the future. Ultimately, he's going to repeat whichever behavior gets him the candy, and for most parents, we'd prefer to teach him to repeat a behavior we like. The same concept applies to children waking us at night. Each time we allow a child to disturb our sleep and each time we give a child recognition for coming to our rooms (whether the recognition is in the form of getting them a drink or putting them back to bed or allowing them to come to bed with us), we are telling the child that her behavior is acceptable and that she should continue to perform that behavior. This same concept applies when children wake us and ask for a stuffed animal and then later wake us again and ask for a nightlight. Each time our children wake us, they are trying to get more and more attention from us, and again, they are going to repeat whichever behavior gets them the most attention. It's our job to teach our children the appropriate ways and times for them to get the attention they desire.

Inappropriate attention seeking by their children is a problem for most parents, and it can be especially difficult to handle when it occurs during the middle of the night when we are half asleep. The first step toward resolving this issue is to identify your limits, ideally during the daytime hours when you are fully rested and there are no emotions affecting your decision. You need to decide how many hours of sleep you need each night and what your "Do Not Disturb" hours will be. You also need to decide what constitutes an "emergency" during which it is acceptable for your child to wake you. Next, you must explain to your child your new rules. Explain that you need extra sleep and that you won't be able to wake up at night to help her. Explain that there are appropriate times for her to ask for your help (like before bedtime) and that there are inappropriate times for her to ask for your help (like when you are asleep). Be prepared for your child to test you on these new rules and to see how many of them you are willing to "bend." Establish consequences for your child should she break any of your new rules, and be 100% committed to enforcing the consequences should your child test your resolve. Next, you'll need to perform some preemptive planning. Before bedtime, get your child a drink of water (or even better, have your child get herself a drink). Make sure your child has enough blankets before she gets into bed. Buy nightlights or leave bathroom lights on so she can go to the bathroom by herself during the night. Explain to her that you love her very much and that you will see her in the morning. Remember that her coming to you at night is a habit which means it may take some practice for her (and you) to break it. This will almost certainly translate into her coming to your bedroom in an "emergency," probably the very first night you institute the new rules. Remember that what she wants (much more than a drink or a blanket) is attention from you, and the key to breaking this habit for both of you is for you to not give her the attention. This will be very difficult for both of you at first. It is common for children to become upset the first time you enforce a new rule. Many children will cry or yell. Many parents will feel guilty when they feel like they are not giving their children everything they want. Don't feel guilty. Ultimately, your sleep is critical. Once you have a full night's sleep and you are fully rested, you and your child will both benefit. Once you have established the nighttime rules and you have explained them to your child, you need to enforce the rules. Besides not giving in to your child's demands, you will need to be prepared to implement the consequences you established at the outset of your new nighttime sleep schedule. A consequence may be as simple as your child giving up five minutes of television for each nocturnal awakening. My son was motivated by the money in his piggy bank, so the consequence for him was paying money from his piggy bank into a jar in the kitchen. We found a progressive payment plan to be the most effective strategy for my son, so he had to pay 5¢ for the first offense, 10¢ for the next offense, 25¢ for the next offense, $1 for the next, $5 for the next, and $20 for the next. After dropping his quarter into the jar, he realized he didn't want to pay any more money, and he started following the rules. We've also established rewards programs in which we gave our kids a sticker for each time they followed a new rule, and once they accumulated enough stickers, they received a prize (ten stickers translated into a candy bar). Enforcing limits or restrictions on your children entering your bedroom for non-emergencies can improve your sleep tremendously, and it may teach your children to respect other rules you set in your home as well. Ultimately, the goal is to control as many events that are affecting our sleep as we can, and children waking us at night is a very controllable cause of loss of sleep that we can address with some effort. If you have difficulties putting a plan into action, seek suggestions from your doctor or other parents or teachers at your child's school. With some focus and some determination, you will be able to improve your night's sleep and your child's sleep as well.

We've talked about bed partner issues, and we've discussed children issues. Now we need to discuss your own issues that wake you up. As described previously, not emptying their bladders completely is a common reason many people wake at night. If you notice that you are getting up frequently to urinate, you may have discovered the cause of your fatigue. As discussed earlier, there are several reasons people wake at night to go to the bathroom, most of which are very treatable. Discussing the problem with your doctor will most likely lead to a solution for both your fatigue and your urinary problems. Are you experiencing leg cramps or restlessness at night that's waking you? These symptoms wake countless people during the night, and often times, the symptoms are caused by very treatable medical conditions like varicose and spider vein disease or mild dehydration. A trial of compression stockings worn during the day, along with some increased water intake during the day, can provide some answers. If the stockings worn during the day improve your nighttime leg symptoms, they are very likely due to vein disease (both varicose veins and spider veins can cause leg cramps and restlessness), and current vein treatments utilizing lasers and medication injections are much more tolerable and effective than the older surgical options you've heard or read about. If your veins are the cause, ask your doctor to recommend a **phlebologist** (a doctor who specializes in treating varicose and spider veins) who can further evaluate and treat your condition. If the increased water intake improves your symptoms, consider starting a daily routine of increased water intake in an attempt to maintain improved levels of hydration. Do you snore excessively at night, eventually waking yourself? This can be a sign of something as simple as large tonsils or something as significant as sleep apnea. If your own snoring is waking you at night, discuss with your doctor the option of having a sleep study performed to evaluate your sleep habits in more detail. Do you have frequent nightmares that wake you? Nightmares can be caused by stressful events that occur throughout the day, or they can be the result of more complex brain chemical imbalances. If you are experiencing nightmares on a regular basis, discuss this with your doctor who might provide you with some treatment options or might refer you to a **psychiatrist** (a medical doctor who treats psychiatric disorders with a variety of techniques including prescription medications) or a **psychologist** (a person, who may or may not have a doctorate degree in psychology, who typically provides counseling services and other treatment options, but who does not typically prescribe medications to treat psychiatric illnesses).

Returning to Sally's diary, we see another episode of prolonged sleep latency, followed by an early-morning awakening. Depending on the remaining entries in the diary, we might be able to identify a pattern that would make finding the cause of Sally's fatigue much easier. Details that are important to our bodies' energy levels can easily be forgotten if we rely on our memories to store those details for later use. That's why an accurate sleep diary in which we write down as many details as possible surrounding various nocturnal events at the times they happen can be so valuable.

Besides the situations we've already discussed, there are other common correlations between unrestful sleep and specific events or activities that can be identified through the use of a sleep diary. For example, a night shift worker can identify the fluctuations in sleep efficiency when he sleeps during the daytime hours compared to when he sleeps during the nighttime hours. **Shift work sleep disorder** is a common cause of poor sleep patterns, and the alteration from a normal sleep pattern is easily identifiable in a sleep diary. From an accurate sleep diary, we can see that, even though we fall asleep quickly after having a couple glasses of wine before bed, we wake three times during the night for unknown reasons. When we compare this to the week we went without any alcohol before bed, we quickly notice that even though it took us longer to fall asleep without the alcohol, we slept through the entire night without waking and we awoke feeling more rested. In a sleep diary, we can see that taking a 30 minute nap during the day is associated with taking 20 extra minutes to fall asleep at night when compared to the days we don't take a nap.

(Naps, by the way, should be included in your sleep diary since they are episodes of sleep.) When you review your sleep diary, if you find that you are repeatedly waking up at night because you are experiencing difficulty catching your breath, you have to be concerned about the possibility of a breathing problem causing your sleep difficulties. Even if you notice that you have multiple, brief awakenings each night for no apparent reason, obstructive sleep apnea has to be considered as a possible cause. The longer period of time you track your sleep habits, the better you will understand what is keeping you from getting a normal night's sleep. I suggest my patients keep their diaries for at least one week, although one month is ideal in case the events are more sporadic (related to menstrual periods or end-of-the-month reports being due). Again, the more information you have, the better you will be able to find the pattern and figure out the cause of your fatigue, and the sooner you will be able to correct the problem and feel well again.

The next piece of information that can be very helpful in investigating sleep difficulties is a **sleep diary kept by another person** who sees you go to sleep. This will most often be a spouse, but a roommate or child could also provide valuable information. The other person will try to describe the events, times, and details of your sleep patterns from his or her perspective. For example, if we look at Sally's sleep patterns through a sleep diary from Fred's perspective, we might see:

Event	Time	Details
Time before bed	10:30-11:30pm	Reading Stephen King book, drinking cup of coffee.
Go to bed	12:00am	Looks a little restless.
Sleep	???	I was already sleeping.
Snoring	1:00-1:30am	Loud snoring. Almost seemed to stop breathing at times.
Awake	2:30am	Woke with me when I went to the bathroom.
Sleep	2:35am	
Restlessness	3:00-3:30am	Tossing and turning, seemed to be having a bad dream.
Awake	6:00am	Darn alarm! I'm tired.

Even though this diary is similar to the previous one, it allows us to hone in on more possible reasons for Sally's sleep difficulties. For example, we confirm our suspicions about the scary book before bedtime. We get a look at snoring that may be related to **obstructive sleep apnea**. Often the bed partner will describe loud snoring or even episodes of choking or gasping for breath when describing the person's episodes of apnea. These events witnessed by a bed partner may be consistent with significant obstructive sleep apnea, but the person experiencing the events may not be aware that they are occurring because she may not wake up to full consciousness during the apneic episodes. In working toward a diagnosis of obstructive sleep apnea, a bed partner's diary can be invaluable. The final diagnosis will still need to be made in the sleep lab, but getting a bed partner's description can guide us in the right direction. In this bed partner diary, we also get some insight into possible **nightmares** causing sleep disturbances. Again, a bed partner may witness periods of extreme restlessness that can correlate with nightmares. Often, the affected person does not remember these dreams once awake. The more information we gather the better, so having an observer keep his or her diary as long as possible will be beneficial.

Now that you have your diary and your bed partner's diary, you need to look through the diaries and see if you can identify any trends or patterns. If you find a likely cause for your poor sleep, try to fix it. Sometimes, even when you identify a cause of your sleep difficulties, it can take several attempts to finally resolve the problem. If you are fairly sure you know why you are not getting a normal night's sleep and you simply can't correct the problem, be creative and ask for help in your search for solutions. Talk to friends and neighbors, and discuss your issues with your doctor. Finding the right solution may be difficult, so you'll need to remember the impact your fatigue is having on your life, and you'll need to focus on what you will do with your new-found energy once your problem is resolved. If you've tried and tried and you can't identify the cause of your fatigue, bring your diaries to your doctor. Often times the information available in a sleep history fits into your doctor's understanding of different causes for fatigue even though it doesn't fit into yours. Furthermore, your doctor may be able to recommend other pieces of information that could help fill in missing details necessary to make the correct diagnosis.

Another source of information you can develop at home, which very likely will give you clues about why you feel fatigued, is an intake diary. An **intake diary** is a record of everything you put into your body in a given day. In this diary, you would include all food and drink, as well as medications and other drugs. With this diary, you will need four columns to gather adequate information. The first column will be the item taken in. The second column will be the quantity of the item. The third column will be the time it was taken in, and the fourth column will contain any comments or descriptions about the item. Sally's intake diary might look like this:

Item	Quantity	Time	Comments
Coffee	1 cup	6:00am	I'm so tired
Bagel and cream cheese	1	6:30am	A little freezer burned
Multivitamin	1	06:45am	Good for me
Coffee	1 cup	7:00am	Off to work
Doughnut	1	7:30am	Cake doughnut
Ibuprofen	2	9:00am	Headache
Hamburger and fries	1	12:00pm	Lunch
Soda	1 can	12:00pm	Lunch
Cough drop	1	2:00pm	Dry throat
Soda	1 can	3:00pm	Break
Soda	1 can	5:00pm	Drive Home
Pizza	2 slices	5:30pm	Dinner
Soda	1 can	5:30pm	Dinner
Coffee	1 cup	10:30pm	Relaxing
Ginkgo	1 capsule	11:30pm	Helps me deal with stress

As is the case with the sleep diary, the more detail available, the more information we have to help us identify any pattern that may exist. Some of the clues we get from this intake diary include the fact that Sally took in seven caffeine-containing beverages (a slow day for some) within a 24-hour period. Not only will the caffeine perform its normal stimulant effect which can cause sleep difficulties, but it is also a **diuretic**—it makes us put more fluid out into our urine than we take in. This means that Sally took in limited amounts of replenishing liquids that are critical for the body to perform its normal functions, so she is likely living in a chronically dehydrated state. In this case, the caffeine may be causing both sleep disturbances and dehydration, both of which can cause fatigue.

Another item in this intake diary that is important to discuss is the multivitamin. The multivitamin noted in the chart is a good idea, in general, but I would encourage everyone to read the labels on the vitamin bottles before buying them. Not all multivitamins are created equal. I will review some of the most important vitamins and minerals you should be looking for in your multivitamin when I discuss treating fatigue in the next section of this book, but for now I will tell you that there is a lot of variability in vitamin and mineral content among multivitamin pills. Some vitamins can make us drowsy directly, and others can adversely affect sleep leading to fatigue more indirectly. Another key point when reading a vitamin label is to realize that serving sizes aren't always the same from one vitamin to the next. Years ago, when my sons were young, we bought a gummy-bear type vitamin for them. The good news was that they loved them, and I had no problem getting my sons to take them every day. I discovered the bad news a few weeks later when I finally looked at the label on the bottle. Not only were there several key vitamins missing (iron, for example, which is one of the main vitamins we try to supplement for children), but also the dose described for kids over four years old was four gummy bears per day (my boys had only been taking one gummy bear per day, so they were only getting 25% of the vitamins and minerals that were listed on the label). Needless to say, I bought a new multivitamin for my kids during our next trip to the store. Again, not all vitamins are created equal. I encourage you to read the labels before you buy any multivitamin.

The next thing we see in Sally's intake diary is the ibuprofen and cough drop. It's possible that Sally is taking these medications because she is developing cold symptoms.   It's also possible that she has undiagnosed chronic **post-nasal drip** or allergies that are giving her headaches and sore throats (as well as causing poor sleep and/or chronic inflammation leading to fatigue). It's also possible the medications are being used to treat the symptoms caused by the caffeine she's been drinking. Caffeine withdrawal headaches are common, especially if Sally normally has four cups of coffee with breakfast and today only had one. In addition, dehydration can give us **tension headaches** and make our mouths and throats feel dry and irritated. In this situation, looking at the frequency and timing of Sally's use of pain medications and cough drops will give us the clues we need to determine if this is a short-term or a long-term issue and if the symptoms being treated are related to any other activities or events that might be causing her problems. There are times when people are more aware of the specific medications they are taking and why they're taking them, and there are times when people get into the habit of taking medications, take them on a routine basis, and stop paying attention to the reasons why they're putting them into their bodies. An intake diary can help us focus on these issues.

As we look more closely at this intake diary, we also see an example of the extremely **poor nutrition** that is so typical in the United States. We are a society that is always on the go. We don't have time to eat well-balanced, freshly-prepared meals. We want, and often need, meals that are quick and easy to make (frozen dinners and carry out food), and these don't always have optimal nutrition. Depending on the calories, vitamins, minerals, and other substances present in the foods we eat, we can cause a tremendous imbalance in the chemicals in our bodies. As a rule, we eat too many calories, too much sodium, and too much fat. There are various opinions about what proper nutrition should look like. Some people feel we should avoid carbohydrates. Other people feel we should avoid fat. Others feel we should avoid red meats. The truth is that there is limited scientific information regarding what the "correct" diet should contain. As a rule, our bodies can overcome a wide variety of dietary habits without any adverse effects. We're amazingly adaptable creatures. Assuming our bodies are functioning normally, we can probably take in a little extra sodium and some extra carbohydrates and some extra fat and some red meat all without any problem whatsoever. Humans are omnivores which means we were built to eat a wide variety of foods, and while we would likely all benefit from eating a few more fresh fruits and vegetables, the particulars of which foods we are eating probably isn't the most important concern.

The primary problem facing Americans, and unfortunately facing us at a younger and younger age, is the quantities of the foods we are eating. Our bodies are very simple organisms when it comes to how we handle the calories we eat each day. If we eat more calories than we burn in a day, we will gain weight; and if we eat fewer calories than we burn in a day, we will lose weight. As human society has advanced, we've made it much easier to get our food—we now head to the grocery store instead of hunting for meat and gathering grain from the fields. This means that we now have access to essentially as much food as we could want, and it takes little energy to obtain that food. When we were a society of hunters and gatherers, we might only have eaten one meal every one or two days, and we might have had to expend great amounts of energy to obtain that one meal. Because humans didn't have a steady flow of food, the ones who survived were those who would eat as much as they could when the food was available, and their bodies would store the extra calories in the form of fat just in case the next meal didn't come along for a while. During the historical period when food was in short supply and hard to obtain, this strategy of eating more than we needed and storing the extra energy for later was a key survival mechanism. Now it causes us to eat as much as we can at three meals each day, and it leads us to snack between meals. In general terms, the success of America as a society has allowed us to work less hard in order to obtain more food which means we are now able to eat more calories and burn fewer calories on a daily basis. This is exactly what has led us to being an obese country. Obesity is one of the greatest risks to our overall health Americans face.   As we struggle to correct this societal problem, we need to focus on reducing our overall caloric intake and increasing our caloric output. In other words, we need to eat less and exercise more. Beyond that general concept, there is very limited scientific knowledge about specific dietary plans. The benefits or detriments of eating certain quantities of certain nutrients are mostly a matter of opinion, so until the definitive research is complete, my general rule of thumb is to eat everything in moderation. To have a better idea of what "moderation" means, we have to start by understanding exactly what we're putting into our bodies. On every food package and for most restaurants, we can get nutritional information about the food we are eating, and for most foods we prepare, we can get this information from the internet. Even if you can't find the exact, specific nutritional information, getting information for a similar food will give you a ballpark idea of what you're eating. On most food labels, there will be a list of ingredients, and there will also be **% Daily Values (%DV)** listed. These % Daily Value numbers are calculated to tell us what percentage of the total recommended amount of each nutrient is contained in one serving of the food you are eating. One of the first steps in this process is to understand what one serving of a particular food is. For some items, a serving is the whole package. For other items, a serving is only 1/4 of a package which means eating the whole package quadruples the calories and %DV listed on the package. Once you know what amount of a particular food is being used to determine the nutritional content of that food, the next concept that must be understood is that the %DV is usually based on a person who needs to eat 2000 calories per day. For many of us, depending on our activity levels, 2000 calories per day may be too much or too little, so the %DV listed may or may not be exactly correct for each of us. Regardless of the exact number of calories your body needs to exist at your ideal body weight, the % listed on the labels and the grams (g) listed for each nutrient should still be relatively close to your particular needs. Reading labels is the only way to know what you're putting into your body. On the labels, there will be a variety of nutrients listed and recommended amounts of these nutrients. As a general rule, trying to stay somewhere around 100% of these recommended amounts each day is a good goal. If you want to know, based on your body's needs and your specific daily activities, the proper amounts of each nutrient you should eat each day, a consultation with a **dietician** is the best way to come to a more specific understanding. Again, ultimately, the goal is to keep your nutrient intake in balance. If our nutrient intake is significantly out of balance, it can leave us feeling fatigued.

As we continue to move through the intake diary, we notice that Sally is taking **ginkgo.** While Sally may be taking the ginkgo to help with her stress levels, it may also be causing some of her sleep difficulties. Every medication we take can have a variety of effects and side effects on our bodies. We will discuss ginkgo in more detail later in the book, but for now I'll just say that ginkgo can increase a person's energy level and impair her sleep patterns. Since every medication has the possibility of causing changes in a person's energy level, we need to evaluate each medication we take each day. The three key variables of a medication to look at are: which medication is being taken, what dose is being taken, and when is the medication being taken? If you're taking a medication (vitamin, herbal supplement) and it has positive effects (it makes you feel better or has some beneficial effect on your overall health) but negative side effects (you feel fatigued during the day), try adjusting one of the three variables. If you're taking the medication in the morning, try taking it at night or vice versa. If you're taking the full dose all at once, try breaking the dose up into two or three smaller doses. If there are other medications that are similar to the one you're taking, try a different medication and see if the benefits remain and if the side effects resolve. Working with your doctor and a pharmacist can help guide some of these decisions, but sometimes, it simply takes trial and error to find the answer.

When looking for fatigue that is possibly being caused by a medication, keep in mind that medications can cause fatigue in two general ways. Some medications give us too much energy leading to poor sleep and subsequent fatigue. Other medications directly cause a decrease in energy level that will be experienced as fatigue. When looking through an intake diary, consider the fact that not all medications act immediately. Some effects can present themselves several hours after taking the medication because it can take that amount of time for the medication to reach its maximum levels in the blood. Other medications take days or weeks or even months to build up to effective levels in a person's blood, so you may need to look back over a longer period of time in order to find a pattern. Another key medication to include in your diary is **nicotine**. Whether it's in the form of cigarettes, chewing tobacco, pipe smoking, cigars, snuff, or whatever other form, and even if it's in the form of second-hand-smoke, nicotine has such profound effects on a person's energy level and sleep habits that it is crucial to include it when tracking things that are being taken into the body. Eliminating nicotine from your life is, by far, one of the best steps you can take toward improving your health in general, but it's not easy. We'll discuss some steps you can take toward quitting smoking later in the book, but for now, I want to point out that nicotine is among the medications you need to track when you're keeping your intake diary.

The same can be said about **illegal drugs**. Whether it's marijuana, cocaine, methamphetamines, heroin, or prescription drugs that were not prescribed for you, drugs have direct and indirect effects on levels of energy and should be included in your intake diary. When considering sharing this information with your physician, it's important for you to know that physicians maintain this information in confidentiality and do not pass it on to law enforcement. In addition, this is vital information for us to have if we are going to understand why you are experiencing the symptoms you are having. I would encourage you to share this information with your physician if you desire to have your symptoms fully evaluated and treated.

When looking through the intake diary, you will want to look for patterns. Do you feel different on the days you drink more or less caffeine? How does taking your medications at different times of the day, or possibly forgetting your medications, affect your symptoms? Are you eating a reasonable range of foods? How do you feel on the days you drink more or less water? Are you taking any medications that you are using to treat side effects from other things you do to your body? As we discussed with sleep diaries, with intake diaries, look for patterns you can identify, and try to fix anything that appears to be causing your symptoms. Try several solutions to see if one adjustment is more effective than another. Finally, if you are not able to identify a pattern or find a workable solution, review your intake diary with your doctor and see if she is able to relate your intake to your symptoms and develop a treatment plan for you.

So far, we've reviewed sleep patterns and intake patterns. The final piece of information you can gather that will help complete the picture of why you feel fatigued is an output diary. An **output diary** should include information about how you spend your time during the day, how much time you spend doing each activity, where the activity is done, the time of day it's done, and any comments you want to make about the activity. If your fatigue comes and goes, the most important observations you can make are related to what you are doing before you notice the fatigue, as well as what you are doing at the time you become fatigued. It's also helpful to track how long the fatigue lasts. Again, detail is helpful, so do the best you can to put as much information as you can into your output diary. For Sally, her output diary might look like this:

Activity	Time of Day	Location	Comments
Get ready for work	6:00-7:00am	Home	I'm tired
Drive to work	7:00-7:30am	Car	
Work	7:30am-5:00pm	Work	I love my job!? I felt particularly tired from 1:00-3:00pm
Drive home	5:00-5:30pm	Car	I love traffic!?
Eat dinner	5:30-6:00pm	Home	In front of TV
Watch TV	6:00-10:30pm	Home	
Read book	10:30-11:30pm	Home	In bed
Get ready for bed	11:30pm-12:00am	Home	I'm so tired!

From this diary we can identify several issues that are common causes of fatigue that could have been overlooked if they weren't written down. First of all, we notice that Sally had a long day, but none of this day was spent burning significant amounts of calories. With **exercise**, our bodies become more efficient—our hearts develop the ability to pump more blood per beat; our muscles learn to utilize energy more efficiently; and our waste

123

disposal systems become more effective at clearing out the waste products. We will discuss exercise in more detail later, but for now, realize that regular amounts of exercise are important for maintaining regular body function and for maintaining normal energy levels.

In an output diary, we might identify activities that we are engaging in that are causing fatigue, and we might find a relative lack of activities (like exercise) that are similarly causing fatigue. Another issue identified in Sally's output diary is the tremendous level of stress involved in her daily life. Work and traffic, among many other situations throughout the day, increase Sally's level of stress. As discussed earlier, stress causes the release of stress hormones leading to the release of inflammatory mediators that can cause us to feel fatigued. Using an output diary can help to identify particularly stressful events in our days. Once identified, we can look for opportunities to reduce stress throughout the day. Whether it's through meditation or reading or exercising or some other activity that helps us relax, finding ways and taking the time to relax will help relieve some of the daily stress and can be invaluable for improving our energy levels. As we discuss ways to improve energy levels, I often review with my patients the benefits of regular exercise as well as the benefits of focused relaxation. When a person comes to me saying they don't have time to exercise because they are too busy (a very common comment in my office), or when they tell me they can't find any more time in the day to relax or to sleep, I ask them what they watched on television yesterday. They usually remember the prime-time shows or sporting events, but the news and movies frequently slip their minds. Besides the time spent watching television, we also have to consider the time spent surfing the **internet** as time that could be spent in alternative ways. For most of us, significant amounts of time are spent each day engaged in activities that have questionable health benefits for our lives. The last I heard, the average American watches more than four hours of television and spends more than two hours surfing the internet each day. While some amount of television or internet usage may be beneficial to help us relax, at least some of the roughly 400 minutes we spend on these activities each day could be exchanged for more productive ones. While watching television and working on a computer, our bodies are relatively inactive, and from the perspective of body metabolism and energy levels, much of this time is wasted. Trading at least 30 minutes (and preferably 60 minutes) each day of television and/or internet usage for exercise can produce impressive results for your physical health, your mental health, and your energy level. Swapping another 10 minutes each day for meditation and an additional 60 minutes each day for sleep will have a miraculous impact on your life. Sometimes, in order to "find" the time for exercise, relaxation, and sleep we need to make a special effort to consolidate and budget our television watching and internet usage. Rather than checking our Facebook accounts for five minutes each time, ten times each day, we can budget a 15-minute Facebook session in the morning and a 15-minute session in the evening. Rather than watching our favorite shows on TV and then sitting in front of the television set as the next couple shows run across the screen, we can plan our evening of TV watching and turn the television off as soon as our shows end. As most people look at their output diaries, they will almost always be able to find more potential free time than they might have initially thought. It's up to each of us to decide how we want to spend that time.

The output diary is the final piece of information you need to help you determine why you are tired. If you can compose all four diaries during the same period of time (again, it should be for at least one week, and a month or more is even better), that's ideal. If you need to work on one diary at a time, that will work. Now that you have all the pieces, the next step is to put the puzzle together. Look at all four pieces of paper. See how you are spending your days. How do the activities of the day and night affect how you feel the next day? Can you find any patterns? If you change one thing in one of the lists, how does it affect the other things in the other lists? Have you figured out why you're so tired? Make changes, and see what effects the changes produce.

Keep tweaking your days in an effort to fine tune your energy level. Again, I encourage you to review your lists with your friends and family members and to bring these lists to your doctor if you can't find a pattern. Each person who looks at your lists may see something different. Your doctor has been trained to look for certain clues when trying to identify the causes of fatigue, so there may be something your doctor might see that you don't, and again, your doctor may be able to point you in the direction of finding the last bit of information necessary to make the diagnosis and institute an effective treatment.

Chapter 7: What Can Healthcare Professionals Do for You?

By the time people make an appointment to see me about their fatigue, they are usually very frustrated and very concerned about what might be going on. Of course, things like cancer and depression are the first things they want me to check them for, but after a little discussion, they soon realize that the causes of fatigue are extremely varied and that there are much more likely causes of fatigue than cancer and depression—none of which are quite as frightening for most of my patients. My first step in discovering the causes of my patients' fatigue is to talk to them. I try to find out if they are experiencing any symptoms that might give me a clue. In some cases, the descriptions people give me of what's been going on, for how long, and in what situations tell me exactly why they're experiencing their fatigue. However, there are still significant numbers of people for whom I don't have an answer after our initial discussion. My next step is to examine the patients. Do their eyes look yellow? Do they look pale? Are they overweight? Do they have signs of chronic allergies or sinus congestion? Do their lungs sound congested? Do their hearts beat normally? Do they have any pain in their stomachs? Do they have any swelling in their legs? Do they answer my questions appropriately? On occasion, I'll find my answer during my examination, but for the remaining folks, we move on to testing.

The remainder of this chapter will be dedicated to descriptions of the types of testing my patients undergo during the workup for their fatigue. There is no particular order to these tests. I will typically perform the test that I think is most likely to give me my answer first, followed by the tests for less and less likely diagnoses. After going through my evaluation and not finding the answer, I will refer my patients to specialists for further evaluation, and, just like with the testing, I start out by referring them to the specialist I think is most likely to give us the answer followed by the specialists for the less and less likely diagnoses. As a reminder, in a small percentage of my patients, even after undergoing extensive testing and several referrals, there is no answer to the cause of their fatigue. In these cases, I reassure them that they really do have something medically wrong with them and that we will try therapies that we use for other diseases until we find a treatment that works. This entire process takes time, so patience and persistence are very important.

Knowing that abnormalities of sleep and activity are the most common causes of fatigue, my first step in evaluating my fatigued patients, if they haven't already brought me the information, is to have my patients keep the four diaries discussed in the last chapter (sleep diary, bed partner's sleep diary, intake diary, and output diary). These sources of information are extremely helpful when I'm looking for clues to the causes of my patients' fatigue. Answers I couldn't find during my interview with the patients often become obvious when reviewing their diaries. Again, sleep abnormalities are remarkably common causes of fatigue, so I typically look very closely at a patient's sleep diary as my first step. If the person has a history of loud snoring or if she frequently wakes up in the morning not feeling refreshed, I immediately begin to suspect obstructive sleep apnea, and one of the first tests I will order will either be an overnight oxygen monitoring test or, more likely, a full sleep study.

During a full **sleep study**, the patient goes to a sleep lab, frequently located in a hospital or some other medical clinic, and spends the night in the lab. During the night, the technologist responsible for monitoring the patient, monitors heart activity, oxygen levels in the blood, movement of the chest, and movement of air through the nose and mouth. Occasionally, we will also monitor brain activity, eye movement, and muscle tone during a sleep study. As you might expect, the technologist needs to connect many wires and sensors to the person in order to measure each of these activities, and while sleeping in a medical lab setting hooked up to all kinds of machinery isn't as comfortable as sleeping at home in your own bed, none of the sleep testing involves anything painful. During a sleep study we can detect numerous abnormalities of sleep. For example, if a sleeping person shows normal or even exaggerated movement of the chest with little or no movement of air through the nose or mouth, this would suggest that the person is trying to breathe but cannot, and this would be consistent with **obstructive sleep apnea**. If the person doesn't make any effort to breathe despite falling oxygen levels, this would suggest the person's brain isn't sensing oxygen levels normally, and this would be consistent with something called **central sleep apnea**. During the sleep study, we can accurately measure the time between lying down and falling asleep (**sleep latency**). We can also measure the number and duration of each of the phases of sleep, and we can identify abnormal sleep architecture. We measure the duration and frequency of episodes of waking up which give clues about other causes for disturbed sleep. Finally, the technologist can make helpful observations about restlessness and body position during sleep. Each of these factors is looked at and compared to a normal sleep pattern and to the person's symptoms to determine if the person has a sleep-related cause for their fatigue. If an abnormality is identified during a sleep study, your doctor will discuss the abnormality with you and make some suggestions about possible ways to improve your sleep pattern. One of the most commonly diagnosed disorders discovered during a sleep study is obstructive sleep apnea, and since this involves the airway closing when a sleeping person is trying to breathe in, the best treatment for obstructive sleep apnea is to apply air to the back of the throat to keep the throat open when the person breathes in. We apply this air to the throat using a mask that goes over a person's nose and/or mouth, and we call this treatment **continuous positive airway pressure or CPAP**. We will discuss CPAP and other treatments for obstructive sleep apnea later in the book, but for now, I want you to understand that CPAP has been an amazing advance in the field of medicine overall and is a very successful treatment for many people who suffer with a variety of symptoms related to obstructive sleep apnea.

There are several challenges associated with performing a sleep study in a sleep lab including the fact that not all towns have easy access to sleep labs, sleep studies are expensive, and people often aren't able to accomplish a "normal" night's sleep (how they typically sleep at home) in a lab setting. Because of these limitations, we are researching the use of home sleep monitoring equipment that would allow a person to sleep in a more natural environment yet still provide the same information obtained from a sleep study performed in a sleep lab. Unfortunately, at this point in time, the equipment is too fragile, and there are too many inconsistencies in the reports we receive to make the information we obtain from home systems as reliable and as useful as that we obtain in sleep labs. This will undoubtedly change in the future, and someday, we will be able to get a comprehensive sleep study from a portable system. If a full sleep study isn't feasible, we can reduce our evaluation to the information we get from a home oxygen monitor. The **home oxygen monitor** measures oxygen levels in a person's blood using a sticker that attaches to the person's finger. The machines are small, portable, and accurate. They are inexpensive and can be brought into a person's home. They provide information about the blood oxygen levels occurring during sleep, and they suggest the presence of sleep apnea or some other diseases (such as congestive heart failure or emphysema) that cause low oxygen levels during sleep. Depending on the availability of a full sleep study, we often begin our evaluation of sleep difficulties with a home oxygen monitor, and, depending on the results, move on to a full sleep study if we need to obtain more detailed information.

The other device we can use at home to help determine the efficiency and duration of sleep is a machine that measures body movement. The machine is called an **actigraph**. This machine measures movement, so while awake, there should be more activity measured, and while asleep, there should be less activity measured.   When we compare measured activity with reported sleep periods in a sleep diary, we can obtain useful information about restlessness during sleep. As with the home oxygen monitor, an abnormal study on an actigraph suggests that there's a problem, but it doesn't tell us exactly what the problem is. So, if the study is normal, we know that the person isn't overly active during sleep, but if the study is abnormal, additional testing will be needed to figure out why.

As we have discussed throughout this book, many of the most common causes of fatigue are directly or indirectly related to abnormal sleep patterns, but there are other causes as well. Besides evaluating sleep, we need to look for abnormalities in the chemicals in the blood to be sure they are not causing fatigue. One of the most important chemicals we check is called **thyroid stimulating hormone (TSH)**.   We discussed the function of thyroid hormone in a previous section of this book.   Thyroid hormone normally circulates throughout the body, including the brain. In the brain, there is a sensor that determines if there is the correct amount of thyroid hormone in the blood. This sensor is connected to a part of the brain that releases another hormone (thyroid stimulating hormone) whose job is to stimulate our thyroid glands to release more thyroid hormone (just to be clear, thyroid hormone and thyroid stimulating hormone are two completely separate hormones that have completely different actions despite the fact that their names are very similar). If the sensor in the brain feels there isn't enough thyroid hormone floating around, it will cause the release of more TSH that should stimulate the thyroid gland to release more thyroid hormone. If the sensor feels there is already enough thyroid hormone present, it will not release as much TSH. If either the sensor or the thyroid gland doesn't work properly, we can end up with an abnormality in thyroid levels. The test available to measure TSH in the blood is much cheaper and much easier to get than the test available to measure thyroid hormone itself, so we usually start by measuring TSH levels. If the TSH level is abnormal, we then will typically move on to measuring thyroid hormone levels directly. Depending on the results, we can determine if the problem is being caused by the brain and its release of TSH or by the thyroid gland and its response to TSH. The most common abnormality is in the thyroid gland which means the brain is releasing extra TSH (so the TSH levels will be elevated), but the thyroid hormone levels themselves will be low. We call this low level of thyroid hormone **hypothyroidism**. In these cases, we typically treat the abnormality by giving extra thyroid hormone in an effort to bring the thyroid hormone levels back to normal. Most often, because each pill is manufactured with very consistent amounts of the hormone, we use a synthetic thyroid hormone (levothyroxine) to treat hypothyroidism. Some doctors prefer to use other forms of thyroid hormone for a variety of reasons, so if you are diagnosed with hypothyroidism, be sure you understand which thyroid medication you are taking and what the advantages and disadvantages are before you start taking the medication. Unfortunately, the thyroid gland may produce varying amounts of thyroid hormone over time, so ongoing TSH levels will need to be measured and adjustments to your supplemental thyroid hormone will likely need to be made periodically.

Among the other blood tests I typically order when I'm evaluating a person with fatigue is a **complete blood count (CBC)**. A CBC provides us with numerous pieces of information about the composition of a person's blood. **White blood cells (WBC)** are part of our immune systems, and they are one of the cells identified in a CBC. If white blood cells are increased or decreased in number, this could suggest an infection. If they are extremely elevated, this might suggest cancer of the white blood cells called **leukemia**. White blood cells have different subtypes (**neutrophils, basophils, monocytes, lymphocytes, and eosinophils**), and each subtype can be above or below normal levels. A variation in either direction from normal can suggest different possible problems, so while measuring the white blood cells in total, we also count the different subtypes of white blood cells. Different types of white blood cells can be increased or decreased depending on what type of immune system stimulation a person has undergone. Some subtypes are increased when we have bacterial infections (neutrophils typically); others are increased when we have viral infections (lymphocytes typically); and still others are increased when we have infections with parasites or funguses (eosinophils typically). Allergic reactions can increase basophils and eosinophils. These relative elevations vary from person to person, so your doctor will review the relative ratio of each component and will discuss with you the most likely significance of the findings. Along these same lines, it's possible to have an infection causing chronic fatigue but to have a normal WBC count and normal numbers of the subtypes. This is more common after an infection has been present for a prolonged period of time and the immune system has "gotten used to" it. This kind of variability in lab results is one of the biggest challenges we doctors face as we try to interpret the information obtained.

The next component of the CBC we look at is the red blood cells. As we discussed earlier, **red blood cells (RBCs)** carry hemoglobin which has the job of carrying oxygen throughout the body. From a CBC we can tell if the red blood cells are of a normal shape and size. We can also measure whether the blood's overall oxygen-carrying capacity (hemoglobin) is normal. We can determine if the blood has the correct volume of red blood cells compared to the total volume of the blood. We can also tell if we are producing the proper number of new red blood cells. These studies can detect a variety of different abnormalities of the red blood cells. They can help us determine if a person has anemia and if so, what the likely cause of the anemia is. Although some other tests of the red blood cells may be necessary to pin down the exact cause of a particular case of anemia, we can often initiate treatment of the disease based solely on the red blood cell findings in a CBC.

The final piece of information available in a CBC regards the platelets. **Platelets** are cells that are used by our bodies to stop bleeding. They are the primary building blocks of scabs and blood clots. From a CBC, we measure the number and shape and size of the platelets, and this information gives us insight into possible clotting disorders. If platelets are too low (called **thrombocytopenia**), there could be a risk of bleeding too easily. A lower-than-normal level of platelets can suggest inadequate production due to a dysfunction of the platelet-producing cells that are located in the bone marrow, and abnormal bone marrow function can be caused by an infection or cancer or a variety of other causes. Increased platelet numbers (called **thrombocytosis**) can lead to an increased risk of blood clot formation. In addition, elevated platelet counts often correspond to the presence of inflammation in the body, and this, along with other lab tests taken at the same time, may lead us to the cause of the immune system activation.

The findings in a CBC can give us many clues to possible causes of fatigue. If the levels of all the components of the blood are elevated, we consider **dehydration** as a possible cause. When all of the components are low, this suggests a possible infection or possible cancer. When one or another component is low or high, numerous interpretations may be suggested. A CBC is a very common test, and we run this test in a wide variety of situations in order to monitor an array of diseases. It's quite amazing the amount of information we can get from such a basic laboratory study. This is a test that will be performed on most people on numerous occasions throughout their lives, and for this reason, I think it's a good idea for patients to understand what information we're looking for when we run it and how this information can be used.

Through our discussion of the various causes of chronic fatigue, we've discussed several that are associated with increased levels of inflammation in a person's body. While there are many chemicals that are part of the inflammatory cascade, two of the chemicals we commonly measure in the blood are the **erythrocyte sedimentation rate (ESR)** and **C-reactive protein (CRP)**. These chemicals are easy to measure; the tests are inexpensive; and the results are available very quickly. Elevated levels of these chemicals suggest that inflammation is present. Unfortunately, these tests don't tell us what's causing the inflammation. As we discussed earlier, an elevated ESR or CRP can be due to a variety of different medical conditions. Elevated levels of these chemicals are simply an indication that we need to keep looking for the cause of the inflammation. Depending on the symptoms present, we might start searching for an autoimmune disease. For example, if the patient has joint pain and swelling, we might consider rheumatoid arthritis as the possible cause of the inflammation. If the patient has a rash, we might be more suspicious of lupus. Unfortunately, many autoimmune diseases have overlapping symptoms, so a particular diagnosis almost always requires a specific constellation of lab tests and physical exam findings before it can be positively identified. Also, many diseases that stimulate inflammation, including autoimmune diseases, go through periods of increased activity (called **flares**) and periods of decreased activity (called **remissions**). Depending on what level of inflammation is present at the time of testing, a person who is in a remission might have a normal ESR or CRP which can be very misleading as we search for the cause of a patient's symptoms. This means that a low level of either of these chemicals doesn't necessarily rule out an inflammatory disease as the cause of the symptoms, but it might encourage us to look towards other possible causes or to recheck the ESR or CRP at a later time. Besides using these tests as screening tools to decide what additional testing is necessary, we also use them to monitor the effectiveness of treatments. Once we've determined that an inflammatory disease is present and once we start treating the disease, we can check the levels of inflammation using the ESR or CRP results over time. These results tell us whether or not our treatment is reducing the inflammation and effectively treating the disease. Measurements of inflammation are very valuable, and they are commonly used by doctors. Because they are so commonly used, it is highly beneficial for patients to understand what they might mean and how they might be used. Also, because there are so many possible meanings and uses for these tests,

135

discussing the results of the tests with your doctor is even more important.

Once we've determined that an ESR or CRP is elevated and if we suspect an autoimmune disease, the next test we might run is an **antinuclear antibody (ANA)**. An ANA measures levels of our body's immune chemicals (called **antibodies**) that have been built specifically to attack the cores of our own cells. (The **nucleus** of a cell is similar to the yolk of an egg in that the nucleus sits inside the middle of each cell. "**Antinuclear**" means the antibodies fight against the nuclei of the cells.) Interestingly, many of us have low levels of these antinuclear antibodies but don't have any symptoms. This means that a slightly positive ANA test may be meaningless. However, once the levels become more significantly elevated, we become suspicious that an autoimmune disease is causing the symptoms. As with an ESR or a CRP, an ANA is a screening test. If the test is positive, it suggests that an autoimmune disease may be present, but it doesn't necessarily tell us which autoimmune disease it might be. In order to make the final diagnosis, your doctor will use the information from the ANA test, along with several other blood tests, possibly biopsies of different areas, and the physical signs present during his examination of you. It's a complex process, so discussing the test results with your doctor will be critical to your understanding of where you stand in diagnosing your possible autoimmune disease.

The final common blood test we send off from my office when looking for a cause of fatigue is a general chemical analysis of the blood, usually called a **comprehensive metabolic panel (CMP)**. This CMP measures levels of a number of chemicals including sodium, potassium, chloride, calcium, glucose, and carbon dioxide. It includes measurements of the kidneys' ability to get rid of waste products as well as a rough determination for dehydration. It gives us information about the liver's health and function and gives us insight into nutritional status—whether the liver has the building blocks necessary to make the proteins our bodies need for daily life. The CMP can tell us if the liver is being irritated by something. Liver irritation can be related to infection of the liver (most commonly the hepatitis infections we discussed earlier) or it can be related to injury of the liver caused by alcohol or medications. As discussed in the previous sections of this book, many of the causes of fatigue are related to changes in these chemical levels. As with some of the other blood tests we've discussed, a CMP is a screening test, and if one of the chemicals measured is out of the normal range, additional testing will likely be necessary to identify the specific cause of the problem.

The blood tests we've discussed so far are the most common tests we run, and they allow us to work toward the diagnosis of some of the most common causes of fatigue. However, at times, we need to move on to the more **unusual blood tests**. These include tests for various infections like Epstein-Barr virus, human immunodeficiency virus, Lyme disease, syphilis, hepatitis B and C, as well as tuberculosis. We can also run tests for unusual chemical imbalances such as abnormalities in the levels of vitamin B12, folate, copper, carbon monoxide, zinc, lead, iron, and magnesium. There are thousands of tests your doctor might order, and different findings in different patterns give us information about the possible diagnoses. Depending on the abnormalities found, we try to select the treatment that is most likely to help the symptoms, but not all treatments work for all people with a particular diagnosis. Again, it's a very complex process that takes time, and patiently working with your doctor through the process is critical.

As we search for possible causes of fatigue, besides blood testing, we may also run **tests on the urine** to make sure the kidneys are functioning properly. We can look for white blood cells in the urine which might suggest kidney or bladder infections. Red blood cells in the urine might suggest damaged kidneys that are leaking blood into the urine. Red blood cells in the urine might also suggest cancer of the bladder or kidneys, or it might indicate the presence of kidney stones. Glucose in the urine suggests the levels of glucose in the blood are too high, and this often correlates with diabetes. Protein in the urine tends to relate to damage of the kidneys that prevents them from reabsorbing protein normally. Kidney damage leading to protein in the urine is most commonly caused by high blood pressure or diabetes, although sometimes the kidneys leak protein for other reasons. We can also measure the amount of water in the urine which depends on how much fluid is running through the kidneys which is directly related to hydration status. As with blood tests, there's a wide array of tests that can be run on the urine, and we typically combine urine test results with blood test results to get the whole picture.

If, in my search for the cause of my patient's fatigue, I've reviewed the sleep diary, the bed partner's sleep diary, the intake diary, and the output diary without finding a likely cause, and if I've performed all the common tests and they've all come back normal, I may start experimenting with common treatment options in an effort to find a satisfactory regimen. If a patient is taking a prescription medication, I may try changing the timing of taking the medication to see if that affects energy levels in any way. At times, I may switch to another similar medication, or I may stop the medication altogether. I will frequently ask my patients to avoid taking any other medications (vitamins, minerals, herbal supplements, and over-the-counter medications) until we figure out what is causing their symptoms. Since many medications take time to leave a person's body, I typically wait several weeks after changing or stopping a medication before evaluating the effects. In general, I try very hard to identify any possible cause of fatigue that might be medication related since medications are frequently the culprits. If the adjustment of the medication had the desired effect, I typically will see a patient a few months later to make sure the improvement is lasting. If the adjustment of the medication was not successful, I move on to the next step.

At this point, since I've usually done everything I can do to investigate my patient's fatigue, I will often refer my patient to specialists who have different training than I do and who might look at the problem from different perspectives and employ different techniques in diagnosing and treating some of the medical problems that can cause fatigue. I will often make a referral to these same people once I make my diagnosis if I feel a specialist has a better range of treatment options available to him for that particular disease.

Some of the most common referrals I make are to doctors who specialize in dealing with diseases of the muscles, joints, nerves, brain, immune system, and endocrine system. A **neurologist**, for example, specializes in detecting and treating disorders of the nerves and brain. Conditions such as seizures, Alzheimer's disease, Parkinson's disease, and pain that I suspect is being caused by irritation of nerves may be most effectively diagnosed and treated by a neurologist. Those that involve pain in joints, inflammation, autoimmune diseases, chronic fatigue syndrome, and fibromyalgia may be best evaluated and treated by a **rheumatologist** since their area of expertise lies in irritation and inflammation within the body. A **physiatrist** or **physical medicine and rehabilitation (PM&R) doctor** is someone who works at helping people with functional limitations return to performing their normal daily activities. These doctors often work with people who have suffered strokes or have been involved in accidents or have other diseases that limit their mobility, and these doctors work to restore as much of the patient's original function as possible. A **pulmonologist** is a doctor who specializes in diseases of the lungs, and he might be able to help with treating diseases like pulmonary hypertension, sleep apnea, emphysema, asthma, and allergies. **Allergists and immunologists** are doctors who specialize in evaluating and treating allergic conditions, so they, too, may help with people with allergies and asthma as well as other diseases caused by inappropriate immune responses to a person's environment. A **cardiologist** specializes in diagnosing and treating diseases of the heart. They often help manage conditions like atrial fibrillation, hypotension, hypertension, congestive heart failure, abnormalities of the heart valves, and issues related to poor circulation. A **psychiatrist** specializes in detecting and treating the chemical abnormalities in the brain that cause changes in thinking or reacting to situations. They can help with things like depression, anxiety, nightmares, and post-traumatic stress disorder. A patient can be referred to an **anesthesiologist** who specializes in relieving pain. Pain clinics can be invaluable in helping those who have chronic pain that causes a cascade of other symptoms including fatigue. An **endocrinologist** is a doctor who specializes in diagnosing and treating abnormalities of the body's hormonal systems, so they would be most helpful with cases of diabetes, excessive steroid production, and thyroid abnormalities. **Infectious disease specialists** are experts in detecting and treating many illnesses caused by infections, and their help is exceptionally useful when we suspect a person's fatigue is being caused by an unusual infection. When a person's legs are bothering her, either because of pain in the legs or cramping at night or restless leg syndrome that is affecting sleep, a **phlebologist** (a doctor who specializes in the diagnosis and treatment of diseases of the veins) is the best person to evaluate the situation. We commonly have a psychologist evaluate a patient to determine if there is a behavioral issue leading to sleep problems or if a stressful situation is causing the patient's fatigue. **Psychologists** are very good at talking to people and listening to them and evaluating how a person deals with various life situations. Psychologists are also trained to look at the types of abnormal life situations a person faces on a daily basis and to suggest methods that may help. A dietician can be very helpful when the fatigue is thought to be related to a problem with a person's diet. **Dieticians** can evaluate what a person is eating, when they are eating, and how much they are eating, and dieticians can make suggestions about ways to improve the nutritional content of the foods people eat. We often recommend a patient be seen by a **massage therapist** who can help reduce muscle tension and help improve relaxation. We may refer a patient to a **chiropractor** or to a **physical therapist** who can evaluate the way a person uses her body to accomplish her daily tasks. Chiropractors and physical therapists are specialists in movement of the body, and they can make suggestions about ways to move more efficiently and less traumatically. They can also provide guidance on exercises to perform to prevent future issues.

These are the specialists I routinely refer my patients to when I am looking for help with diagnosing and treating more complex cases of chronic fatigue. The descriptions I used above for each of these specialists are generalizations, and the testing and treatment offered by any particular specialist can be much different than I've described above and some of their functions and areas of expertise can overlap. My goal in describing the various specialties is to simply point out that there is a tremendous range of people who can help diagnose and treat fatigue, and sometimes, moving on to the right specialist can be a critical step in feeling normal   again.

What Can Healthcare Professionals Do for You?

Section III: Feeling Good Again

Feeling Good Again

Chapter 8: The Basics

Having arrived at this point in the book, I expect one of two things has happened. Either you now understand why you feel the way you do and are ready to correct whatever it is that is causing your fatigue, or you still don't know exactly why you are fatigued but you are ready to make some changes in your life that are likely to make you feel normal again. In this section of the book, I will describe some of the basic steps you can take at home that can increase your energy level and leave you ready to take on everything life places in front of you. These suggestions are good, basic, normal routines you can become accustomed to, yet they can have profound effects on how you feel.

As you can imagine, it all begins with sleep. I can't emphasize enough the importance of getting a full amount of normal sleep each night. We all have different internal clocks, so the exact number of hours of sleep each one of us requires can vary (it's probably somewhere between six and ten hours each night), but if you are tired, there is a very good chance that the amount of sleep you are getting isn't adequate for your internal clock. To correct this, you need to provide yourself with every opportunity for a good night's sleep. First of all, you must schedule yourself for enough sleep time each night. Start off by looking through your sleep diary and seeing how many hours you are in bed each night. If it's less than six hours, I suggest scheduling at that much time. If you're in bed at least six hours each night and are still feeling fatigued, I suggest you add time to your sleep schedule. As a starting point, you can add an hour to each night's sleep (so if you've been in bed for six hours each night, try seven; if you've been in bed for eight hours each night, try nine). It may take a week or so before you feel the effects of the increased amount of sleep time, so wait that long after each increase in sleep time before measuring the effect. If you feel normal with the added time, keep it in your sleep schedule. If you still feel fatigued, add another hour each night. Keep adding time until you feel like you have a normal amount of energy or until you get to ten hours of sleep each night. Very few people require more than ten hours of sleep each night, so if you're in bed for ten hours each night and are still feeling fatigued, the number of hours scheduled for sleep is less likely to be the problem. Scheduling this time into your day may mean that you will be forced to give up some of your other daily activities. As we discussed earlier, once you've performed an output diary, you'll have a good idea of how you spend your time each day and where you might be able to get some extra time for sleep. In the long run, imagine how much more you will be able to get done during your waking hours when you have a normal amount of energy. Rather than dragging through each day, you will be moving through each day at full speed. Ultimately, I am certain that any activity you give up in your effort to increase your sleep will be well worth it, and I suspect you will end up getting much more done each day even though you will have spent more time in bed.

After you've set aside the correct amount of time for sleep each night, the next step is to evaluate what percentage of your time in bed is spent actually sleeping. Very few of us have perfect sleep efficiency, so even if we schedule eight hours of sleep for the night, it is unlikely that we will get a full eight hours of actual sleep. The best way to improve sleep efficiency is to avoid the things we know interfere with it. One part of this is practicing good **sleep hygiene**. As we discussed before, good sleep hygiene includes sleeping during the hours that are meant for sleep and not sleeping during other. The simplest step you can take to achieve this goal is to avoid taking naps. There is no better way to alter your body's sleep cycle than to sleep during the time of day that you should be awake. When you take a nap, your brain is tempted to be awake during the time you should be asleep. Good sleep hygiene also means that if you wake up at 2:00am and you can't fall back asleep within a short period of time (20 minutes or less), get up and try to resolve whatever issues woke you. Often we wake up during the night because we have things on our minds.

We start thinking about the big meeting tomorrow, or we try to figure out how we are going to squeeze all of the items on our to-do lists into the limited amount of time we have. Getting up when you can't sleep allows your brain to process whatever thoughts are running through it. When you're tired again, go back to sleep. Hopefully, once you have dealt with whatever's on your mind, you will be able to return to good sleep for the remaining amount of time you have scheduled for it. Remember that you may be tired the next day. Be patient and keep in mind that you are making an investment in your sleep future. If you can learn to sleep only at night, when you are tired, you will soon train your brain to sleep more effectively when it has the chance. Staying awake when you are not tired and not sleeping at the times you shouldn't be will force your brain to be more fatigued and more accepting of sleep when the chance is given. Only offer your brain the chance to sleep at night, during the time you have set aside for sleep. Good sleep hygiene also includes avoiding the other pitfalls that typically disrupt a normal-night's sleep. For example, in order to avoid confusing your brain, bed should primarily be a place to sleep. Watching television or reading in bed sends a mixed signal to your brain—sometimes you go to this place when you want to sleep and sometimes you go to this place when you want to stay awake. Reserve your bed for sleep alone, and you'll find your brain will become accustomed to falling asleep as soon as your head hits your pillow. By the same token, when you are tired and ready to go to sleep, you should go to your bed. I frequently see people who like to fall asleep in their favorite chairs. The problem with sleeping in the chair is the same as the problem with reading or watching television in bed. We usually use our favorite chairs not only for sleep but also to read a good book or watch television. Again, this sends mixed messages to our brains. I suggest you reserve you chair for reading and watching television. If your chair is more comfortable than your bed, buy a new mattress. If your chair helps you sleep more upright because you can't sleep flat in your bed, put wooden blocks under the head of your bed frame or sleep on more than one pillow in order to raise your head while you sleep (also discuss these symptoms with your doctor because there is possibly some other medical problem that needs to be corrected). The sooner your brain learns that your bed is a place for sleep, the sooner you will improve your sleep efficiency, and the closer you will be to feeling rested in the morning.

Now that you've set aside enough time for sleep and you've trained your brain that your bed is a place to sleep, you need to reduce or eliminate the external events that wake you at night. Fix the simple things first, and fix them before you get into bed. If you find you get cold at night, put extra blankets on your bed. If you get too hot at night, put fewer blankets on the bed or have a small fan blowing on you when you sleep. If there's too much noise in your room, wear ear plugs to bed. If there's too much light in your room, wear a sleeping mask at night. If your bed partner keeps you awake due to snoring or restlessness or going to bed too late or waking too early, think about using ear plugs and a sleeping mask for sleep. Perhaps your bed partner needs some help with his sleep issues which would improve his energy level and yours. Sometimes a low-motion bed can reduce the amount of movement you feel when your bed partner tosses and turns. Sometimes, separate mattresses are the best solution. If all else fails, think about sleeping in a separate room from your bed partner. Your health is very important, and if you don't feel well, you won't be very good at providing the care and compassion that are necessary for a healthy relationship. If your children repeatedly wake you during the night, have a talk with them and let them know that you need your sleep and that they shouldn't disturb you at night. If that doesn't work, consider ignoring them or locking your door at night while you sleep. Rarely do children wake you during the night for true emergencies. Usually, whatever issue was important at 2:00am will still be there at 7:00am. While it may be traumatic at first, children will learn that your sleep time is important, and typically, after a couple unsuccessful trips to your room, they will learn to stay in their own beds for the whole night which will lead to improved sleep for both you and your children. The final step in improving your sleep efficiency is to avoid things that are likely to disrupt a normal night's sleep. Don't drink caffeine in the evening (for some folks, caffeine's effects can last up to six hours, so consider avoiding all caffeine after dinner). Avoid alcohol before you go to bed (alcohol's effects typically last up to four hours). Don't read that thought-provoking book or watch that intense movie just before you try to fall asleep. Save them for daytime hours, or be sure to put some relaxation time between them and trying to go to sleep. If you are too mentally alert to fall asleep, take a hot shower or a bath or meditate before going to bed. Most people do not achieve maximal sleep effectiveness. Many of us do not spend enough hours asleep. Some people's brains can overcome this shortcoming, but the majority end up feeling chronically fatigued. Improving your sleep habits is, without exception, THE best step you can take towards resolving your difficulties with fatigue, so make it a top priority.

Once you get started on improving your sleep habits, the next step is to increase your body's efficient use of its energy supply. The goal is to give your body a steady supply of calories to fuel your day's activities. When we eat foods that have large amounts of simple sugars (whether it's white sugar, brown sugar, honey, or fructose in fruit or fruit juice) or when the foods have large amounts of processed carbohydrates in them such as white bread or white rice, our digestive systems break these foods down very quickly which results in a burst of energy. This is either used or stored very quickly which means there is less energy available for use later. This may translate into feeling fatigued when the burst of energy wears off, or it could stimulate us to eat more food at that point. Neither situation is healthy for us. By the same token, if we eat foods that only contain protein or fat or complex carbohydrates, it takes time to break these foods down into glucose, so there may be a delay between the time we eat and the time we begin to benefit from the energy we just took in. This delay may cause us to want to eat more now in an effort to increase our current energy levels, or it may lead to a delay in the start of our utilization of the energy. Again, this isn't an ideal scenario. If we want an immediate boost of energy and a sustained supply of energy, we should eat meals that have a variety of energy sources in them. We need some simple or processed carbohydrates, some complex carbohydrates or whole grains, some fats, and some proteins in order to provide an even and consistent level of energy for our bodies to use. Eating several (let's say six) smaller meals each day is more likely to provide us with a consistent flow of energy compared to eating two or three meals each day. However, we only need so many calories each day, so if we start to gain weight, it means we are taking in more energy than we are using. In this case, we either need to take in less energy or put out more energy. Obesity is a problem that is affecting more and more Americans every year, and the problem is developing at a younger and younger age. Obesity causes serious health problems including diabetes, high blood pressure, high cholesterol, heart attacks, and strokes. Obesity and fatigue commonly go hand in hand, so fixing one problem will often fix the other. The definition of **obesity** is based on our **body mass index (BMI)**. BMI is calculated from our height (in meters) and our weight (in kilograms). There are plenty of BMI calculators on the internet, but if we want to calculate our own BMI, we can use the following formula. To convert pounds and inches into a BMI we take our weight in pounds and multiply it by 691. We then take this answer and divide it by our height in inches. We finally take that answer and divide it by our height in inches again (so we're dividing by our height twice). Mathematically, this looks like:

$$BMI = \frac{\text{Weight in Kg}}{(\text{Height in meters})^2} = \frac{\text{Weight in lbs x 691}}{(\text{Height in inches})^2}$$

If this number is greater than 30, we are considered to be obese, and weight loss would be an important means of improving our fatigue and our overall health including reducing our risk of developing long-term medical complications. A number between 25 and 30 is considered to be overweight, and weight loss is still recommended. A normal BMI is between 18.5 and 25, and a BMI below 18.5 is considered to be underweight which can be a sign of malnutrition. Historically, we might have looked at someone and suggested that they had a large frame or were "big boned," and this might have led us to suggest a higher weight was healthy for that person; however, the majority of recent research has found a direct correlation between the risk of developing medical complications (diabetes, high blood pressure, high cholesterol) and BMI. While BMI may not be perfect (it may not work for a bodybuilder whose extra weight is all in muscle), it does work for most of us.

If a person's BMI is above 25, and definitely if it's above 30, that person needs to lose weight. The basic concept of **weight loss** is simple—burn more calories than you eat. But in real life, this is a very challenging concept to live out. Unfortunately, there are no shortcuts and no quick fixes. Despite the claims you may read on the internet or see in magazines, there are no magic pills or secret ingredients, and there are no wonder diets that lead to weight loss without effort. Selling weight loss supplements and diet books and aids is a multibillion-dollar industry, and most of these programs are sold with limited research and limited likelihood of providing you with the result you are looking for. In my experience, which is consistent with current research, programs that emphasize restricting caloric intake and increasing caloric output are the most successful means of achieving initial weight loss and maintaining that weight loss in the long run. Overcoming the habit of overeating is one of the most difficult components of reducing caloric intake. For some people, eating a diet high in protein and low in carbohydrates may establish a mental barrier to eating too many calories. For others, eating a diet low in fat may help them avoid eating some of the foods that contain large numbers of calories. For those who eat out of pure habit or who eat in response to stress, looking for ways to break the habit or deal with the stress can be important. Be aware that starving yourself (eating only one or two meals each day or eating less the 1000 calories per day) will stimulate your body's protective mechanisms designed to keep you from starving to death. In these situations, your metabolism will slow down, and you'll have less energy and find it more difficult to lose weight. Eating controlled amounts of food at regular intervals is always a better way to eat. Regardless of the situation, following a specific program helps improve your chances of success, and working through the program with someone else helps with the motivation to follow the program and provides support during the times when you're tempted to take a break from the program. In comparative studies, the program that has been proven to be the most successful, both with initial weight loss and with long-term weight maintenance, is Weight Watchers. Not only do they focus on controlling caloric intake and output, but they also can help with improving the bad habits we've developed over the years, and they provide a support network that enhances the likelihood of success. Weight loss and maintenance are critical for our health. The key is actually how well a person is able to maintain their weight loss over a lifetime rather than over the six months after starting a diet. This means that slow weight loss is just as good as fast weight loss and that changing lifelong habits and continuing those new habits should be the focus. When choosing a diet, you need to choose one you can see yourself continuing to follow for the rest of your life. If you think you'll only be able to "stand" the diet for a few weeks or months, look for another option. Also adding daily exercise to your routine will burn more calories and help you maintain your desired weight. As far as weight loss is concerned, exercise doesn't have to be intense to be beneficial. Going for a walk every day can improve your health, and as time goes on, increasing your exercise intensity can help keep you fit. The goal is to improve your overall health, and healthy eating and routine exercise are the keys to achieving this goal. If you don't know how to get started or if you desire a more personalized plan, consider meeting with a dietician, and consider hiring a **personal trainer** to help you plan your daily workouts. If you have questions about diets and exercise, discuss them with your doctor. Your doctor will most likely be thrilled to discuss your renewed interest in improving your health.

Along with food, we need water, and when I say "water," I mean any substance that contains water. To some extent, this water enters our bodies through the food we eat, but most of it comes from the beverages we drink. As long as our drinks don't contain caffeine or alcohol, our bodies should be able to absorb and retain most of the water from those drinks. As we discussed earlier, the average person needs to drink roughly six cups of water each day in order to maintain a normal level of hydration, and more water is usually better. For some people, it's difficult to drink this much liquid. For others, it's not an issue. One of the major pitfalls I see in my office is that, even though some people drink enough caffeine-free, alcohol-free beverages during the day, their favorite beverages are fruit juices, sodas, and milk. Since juice, soda, and milk have high calorie contents, drinking large volumes of these tends to increase the daily caloric intake, and since most folks don't think of drinks as having calories, people who drink increased amounts of these beverages may start gaining weight and not understand why. Unfortunately, many people think that juice and milk are "good for you," and they forget to consider that these drinks have a lot of calories. While milk and juice do have some nutritional benefits, keep in mind that our bodies can only use so much energy in a day, and whatever energy is left over is stored as fat. Diet, caffeine-free sodas may be fine sources of hydration, but there is ongoing concern and controversy about the safety of some of the chemicals used in these drinks. The same concerns exist for flavorings that we can add to water that improve taste. For these reasons, plain old water is probably the best and the safest way to maintain hydration. Unfortunately, not everyone loves the taste of plain old water, and since dehydration is so common and has such profound effects on our bodies, finding whatever way you can to maintain proper hydration should be your primary goal.

Along the lines of efficient energy usage, our bodies can become more efficient the more they are used. Our hearts, lungs, and muscles are capable of improved functioning with exercise, and the more regularly we exercise, the more efficient they become. When choosing an exercise program, the greatest chance of success comes when you select an activity you enjoy. The more you enjoy it, the more likely you will be to continue exercising every day, and daily exercise is what provides our bodies with the most benefits. For some people, the exercise program includes weight lifting. For others, the best program is in the form of taking the dog for a walk. For some people, exercising at home is the best option. For others, going to the gym and working out with friends is more motivating. Some people hire personal trainers to develop an individualized exercise program. Others focus on daily activities at home like taking laundry up and down stairs and working on landscaping projects. Again, the key is that you find something you enjoy. From a total body efficiency perspective, the most complete types of exercise are **aerobic exercises**. In other words, if you have to breathe heavily and you feel like your heart is beating fast while you are exercising, you are probably providing your body with the type of exercise it needs. Ideally, you should engage in approximately 30 minutes of this type of exercise every day in order to achieve the maximal benefits. If you can't manage 30 minutes each day, start with ten minutes per day, three days per week, and work your way up. If you really enjoy the activity, you will most likely have a hard time limiting yourself to just ten minutes, and the time you spend exercising will increase over time automatically. The most important part of beginning any exercise program is to simply start. Pick an activity and start doing it, even if it isn't the perfect activity and even if it isn't the best workout for the long run. Once you decide to start exercising, you may need to find time somewhere in your daily schedule. Similar to making adjustments in order to ensure enough time to sleep each night, you may need to move things around and budget some of your other daily activities in order to fit in the daily exercise routine. Fortunately, 30 minutes isn't that long a period of time, and for many of us, we can easily exercise and watch television, read a book, or listen to music at the same time. Scheduling some form of exercise into your daily routine is one of the easiest ways to improve your body's metabolism and increase your overall energy level.

The final basic step you can take to ensure your body has the opportunity to function normally is to take in a full complement of vitamins and minerals each day. This can be accomplished in one of two ways. One way is to eat a wide variety of foods and monitor the nutrient content of each food you eat. The second method, and the one I recommend because it's easy (which makes it more likely that people will follow it on a daily basis for the rest of their lives), is to take a **multivitamin**. In my review of the research that has been done on the subject, there is extremely limited scientific evidence suggesting that any one vitamin or mineral is the key to feeling good or that one vitamin form or brand is superior to another. This means that liquid vitamins are just as good as tablets, and inexpensive vitamins can be just as good as expensive ones. The nutritional supplement market is another multibillion-dollar industry, and there is no FDA oversight and no independent company that researches the many claims that are made by the nutritional supplement manufacturers. This means the best thing you can do is to read the labels and be an informed consumer. Here is what a sample label might look like:

Supplement Facts

Serving Size 1 Tablet

	Amount Per Serving	**%DV**
Vitamin A	5000 I.U.	100%
Vitamin C	90 mg	150%
Vitamin D	400 I.U.	100%
Vitamin K	28 mcg	35%
Chloride	7.5 mg	Less than 1%
Boron	150 mcg	*
* % DAILY VALUE (DV) NOT ESTABLISHED		

There are a few general items you can look for when you are reading the label on your next bottle of multivitamins. All multivitamin bottles will list the percent daily value (%DV) of different nutrients contained in one dose of the multivitamin. For some multivitamins, a dose may be one tablet. For others, a dose may be two tablets twice daily (four tablets total) or more. Be sure you know how many tablets you need to take in order to consume the listed %DV. For some nutrients, there is no recommended %DV. This typically means that there is less known about these nutrients and less proven benefit in supplementing them. For example, if the recommended amount of a certain mineral is 100mg and the multivitamin dose contains 10mg, the single multivitamin dose contains 10%DV of that mineral. Ideally we want to get 100%DV of each vitamin and mineral into our bodies each day. This would mean that we would have to take ten doses of this particular multivitamin in order to get a full day's amount of this mineral. For many people, taking ten multivitamin pills each day can become frustrating and expensive. This is one key area where a good quality multivitamin can be helpful. If we can find a multivitamin that has 100%DV of the key vitamins and minerals in one pill each day, most people will find it easier to take that one pill each day, and they will be more likely to continue taking the multivitamin indefinitely (again, lifelong habits are our goal). The %DVs are based on recommendations from the Food and Drug Administration (FDA) about the quantities of each of these vitamins or minerals that seem to be beneficial for our bodies. The exact quantities of the various vitamins and minerals (**mg=milligrams, mcg=micrograms, I.U.=international units**) that equal the amount recommended by the FDA can change from time to time, so it's more important to look at the %DV, rather than the exact quantity, when deciding whether or not you're getting the correct amount of a particular vitamin or mineral. 100%DV will always be the full amount recommended by the FDA. With some medical conditions, your body may need more or less of a certain vitamin or mineral, so if you have questions, always discuss your particular medical situation with your doctor to be sure you know what you need. In general, however, the goal is to take the full

100%DV of each listed vitamin and mineral each day. Taking more than 100%DV of a particular vitamin or mineral generally produces limited benefits, and it may or may not have side effects. Furthermore, the foods we eat contain numerous vitamins and minerals, so, unless you eat an extremely restrictive diet, you will be providing yourself with some amounts of many of the nutrients you need with the foods you eat. You can double check the nutrient content of the foods you eat through a variety of different print and online references (http://www.nutrition.gov/whats-food/vitamins-minerals is a great resource), or you can work with a dietician to make the determination. At the end of each day, your goal should be to have taken in roughly 100%DV of the all the key vitamins and minerals, between your food and your vitamin supplement. How do you decide whether you should buy a multivitamin with 10%DV or 50%DV or 100%DV of certain vitamins and minerals? It depends on your diet. If you eat a wide variety of foods that contain high levels of a variety of vitamins and minerals, a multivitamin with 50%DV should do the trick. If your diet isn't as varied, or if you're not sure what quantities of various vitamins and minerals are in the foods you eat, lean toward a multivitamin that has 100%DV of the key nutrients. In general, it's better to be slightly over the daily recommendations rather than under them. When in doubt, talk to your doctor about your specific situation.

Now that we've finished reviewing the general concepts of vitamin and mineral intake, let's look at some of the specific vitamins and minerals that are most important to our bodies. As we consider people's needs for vitamins and minerals, there are some that are more commonly deficient in our diets than others. In other words, there are some vitamins and minerals that we need to be sure we are adding through supplements. Vitamin **B12** and **iron** are among the most important nutrients to have in a multivitamin. These two nutrients are critical for **hematopoiesis** (red blood cell production), and since iron-deficiency anemia affects up to 5% of the U.S. population and is one of the most common diseases that can be corrected by vitamin supplements, ensuring adequate iron intake through multivitamins is a key step you can take to improve your health. Anemia is especially common in the elderly, in children, in pregnant women, and in menstruating women, so people who fit into these categories should be extra vigilant about taking at least 100%DV of vitamin B12 and iron supplements. Be aware that it is possible to get very sick if you take in too much iron (called **iron toxicity**), but it takes several hundred %DV to get to the toxic dose. The most common situation in which we see iron toxicity is in children who like the taste of their multivitamins. If a child is able to open the bottle of his chewable multivitamins and then eats them like he would a handful of candy, the child can ingest a potentially toxic dose of iron. For this reason, parents need to be very careful with how they store chewable multivitamins. With that said, a correct dose of iron-containing multivitamins remains one of the most important supplements for children to take on a daily basis in order to reduce their risk of developing iron-deficiency anemia. Vitamin D and calcium are the next most important nutrients that should be supplemented. As much as 42% of the U.S. population may be vitamin D deficient even though many of the foods we eat are supplemented with it (especially milk) and even though our bodies can generate vitamin D through exposing our skin to sunlight. As we discussed earlier, activated vitamin D is required for the intestines to absorb calcium, and if inadequate vitamin D and calcium intake lead to low levels of calcium in the blood, the body may start to "steal" calcium from the bones. If enough calcium is stolen from the bones, they eventually become fragile and prone to breaking (bone fragility is called **osteopenia** in the early stages and **osteoporosis** in the late stages). Broken bones in the spine (called **compression fractures** of the vertebrae) and broken hip bones are the two most common types of bone injury caused by osteoporosis. Unfortunately, bones only grow and become stronger when we're young, and they eventually stop growing. For most people, bones are their strongest (also referred to as their peak **bone mineral density** or **BMD**) at age 30, and they become progressively weaker after that time. For this reason, our goal is to build the strongest bones possible by age 30, and to achieve this goal, vitamin D and calcium supplements are important when we're young. We also want the bones to weaken as slowly as possible, so these supplements are important as we age as well. Hormone levels also affect bone mineral density, and women who go through menopause have an accelerated rate of bone loss. This makes it especially important for women (and this includes young women) to supplement their daily vitamin D and calcium intake both before and after menopause. Men can develop osteoporosis, too, and osteoporosis and osteoporotic fractures in men are often ignored. For this reason, men (both young and old) should supplement their calcium and vitamin D intake as well. This means that, as we search for a multivitamin to buy, we need to be sure it has at least 100%DV of both **calcium** and **vitamin D**. The final vitamin I want to specifically discuss in this section is folate. **Folate** (or **folic acid**) is a nutrient our bodies use to build and maintain **DNA** (DNA is the blueprint our cells use to guide the construction of each cell in our bodies). This means that we need adequate amounts of folate in order to ensure new cells are built correctly, and this is especially important when we are growing and developing. For most of us, there are adequate levels of folate in our diets; however, for a developing baby, the amount of folate it receives is determined by its mother's folate intake during pregnancy, and a developing baby needs a much higher amount of folate than other people do. For this reason, folate is one of the most crucial nutrient supplements that a pregnant mother needs to increase during her pregnancy in order to prevent birth defects in her baby. Unfortunately, most women don't always know they're pregnant until several weeks into the pregnancy at which point many parts of the baby have already been formed (either correctly or incorrectly). Because of this delayed recognition of pregnancy, most women who are of child-bearing age should also increase their folate intake during the years that pregnancy is a possibility.

We just spent a fair amount of time reviewing the key nutrients you want to look for when choosing your next multivitamin. Beyond these few vitamins and minerals, there really isn't much consistent evidence for the benefits of the other components of most multivitamins. There may be 20 other ingredients in a multivitamin, and unfortunately, we don't know for sure if they are necessary or beneficial. We often see one research study claim there's a benefit for some supplement, and a short while later, another study finds no benefit. The conflicting results don't mean the situation is hopeless. They merely say that, today, the consistent proof isn't there. I want to emphasize the point that, in general, excess vitamins and minerals don't do any harm. For the most part, they just pass through our bodies without having any effect. If you have been taking a multivitamin for some time that has some specific extra ingredient and you feel better when you take it, keep taking it. Someday, we may discover that the extra ingredient really is beneficial for all people to be taking. On the other hand, if you are new to multivitamins, look for the limited ingredients I've pointed out above. Look for a multivitamin brand you trust. And most importantly, start taking a multivitamin every day. Getting started on a good habit is the hardest part, and improving your nutrition will pay dividends for years to come.

Chapter 9: Other Treatment Options

If you've gone through the basic treatment steps outlined in the previous chapter and you are still feeling fatigued, it's time to start looking at other ways of increasing your energy level. At this point, if you haven't seen your doctor, you need to make an appointment. Your doctor may or may not find the cause of your fatigue, but the chance of it being something more complex increases dramatically once you know that you aren't responding to the treatments that improve the most common causes of fatigue. In this chapter, I will review some of the medications that are commonly used to help with fatigue. I will explain how these medications work, if they work, and some of the potential side effects associated with them. This is by no means meant to be a comprehensive list of medications used to help fatigue, but it includes those most commonly used and even some that are less commonly used. Before taking any of these medications, you should discuss with your doctor or pharmacist whether they might have any significant adverse effects in your particular medical situation. For example, if you have high blood pressure, anxiety, insomnia, or a host of other medical conditions, you may want to avoid some of these medications. It is always safest to ask your doctor before you start taking them rather than after you experience complications due to them.

The first medication I will touch on (because just about everyone uses or has used it at some point in his or her life to help with fatigue) is caffeine. **Caffeine** and its equivalents are present in coffee, tea, soda, and chocolate as well as in commercially-prepared tablets and capsules. Because it's present in such a wide variety of foods and drinks, most of us take in at least small amounts of caffeine or its equivalents periodically throughout our lives. The primary effect of caffeine is an increase in mental alertness which is the effect most people are seeking when they drink their morning coffee. The most common side effects of excessive caffeine intake are increased heart rate, increased blood pressure, jitteriness, nervousness, and intestinal upset including diarrhea. As we discussed earlier, another potential side effect is related to the fact that caffeine can act as a diuretic which can lead to dehydration, so the more caffeinated beverages we drink each day, the more cups of water we need to drink in order to maintain an adequate level of hydration. One aspect of routine caffeine intake that is not commonly acknowledged is the fact that our bodies can become accustomed to caffeine which can translate into less mental alertness from the same dose of caffeine if we keep using it routinely over time. That's the reason the same cup of coffee each morning may or may not provide you with the same effect. Another aspect of caffeine that is often overlooked is that, if we've been consuming caffeine (and it doesn't have to be a large amount) on a regular basis, we can develop withdrawal symptoms (with headache being one of the most common) when we miss a dose. We also need to be cautious because caffeine can make arteries spasm, reducing blood flow to some parts of the body. This is a particular problem for pregnant women (caffeine may reduce blood flow through the placenta to the baby) and for people with heart conditions. For this reason, these people should limit their caffeine intake or avoid it all together. As a reference, an average cola drink has roughly 30mg of caffeine in it; an average cup of coffee has roughly 120mg of caffeine; an average cup of tea has roughly 30mg of caffeine equivalent in it; and an average chocolate bar has roughly 10mg of caffeine equivalent in it. Used sparingly (one to four drinks per day) caffeine and its equivalents can be used to combat fatigue throughout the day, but don't forget the effects on sleep. Caffeine and its equivalents typically take about one hour to start working in your body, and the effects can last 5-15 hours after you ingest it, depending on your metabolism. That means that, depending upon how your body processes caffeine, if you have your morning cup of coffee at 9am, you could still be feeling the effects 15 hours later which would mean you could have a difficult time falling asleep before midnight. The best way to track caffeine's effects and side effects on your body is to compare your intake diary with your sleep diary looking for patterns of time and quantity of caffeine intake compared to sleep efficiency. For most people, the duration of action of caffeine is less than 15 hours, so drinking a cup of coffee in the morning doesn't typically impact that night's sleep. This means that most people can take a dose of caffeine in the mornings on the days they need a little extra mental alertness, and they will likely stay more awake and alert throughout those days without adverse effects on their sleep. You may need to adjust the dosage and timing of your caffeine intake until you become familiar with the effects caffeine can have on your body. As always, watch for side effects, and discontinue use if the side effects are particularly bothersome. Be aware that tolerance and withdrawal can develop quickly, probably within a few days of routine use; so you may need to increase your dose in order to receive the same effects, and when you stop taking the caffeine, you will likely develop a headache. As with any medication, discuss any questions or concerns about your specific medical situation, as it relates to caffeine, with your doctor.

Just like caffeine, **nicotine** is another stimulant medication, and it has essentially the same effects and side effects as caffeine. Because you inhale nicotine into the lungs or because you absorb it through the wall of the mouth, the drug enters the blood stream more quickly that absorbing it through the intestine. Due to the fast rate of absorption, the effects of nicotine are felt much more rapidly than those of caffeine—most people feel the effects of nicotine within a few seconds of taking it into their bodies. Compared to caffeine, nicotine tends to persist in the blood stream for a much shorter period of time (typically only an hour or two) which means that your body will start to feel the effects of withdrawal not too long after taking a dose. Therefore, you will need to use it more frequently in order to maintain the same level of mental alertness from nicotine compared to caffeine. Because the nicotine levels in a person's body rise and fall so rapidly, leading to faster, more frequent episodes of withdrawal, nicotine is much more addictive than caffeine and is probably one of the most addictive drugs sold. These issues make nicotine a less-than-ideal drug to use to help increase energy and alertness; however, the biggest problem with nicotine is the fact that most methods of ingesting it involve taking in other toxic chemicals at the same time. Whether it's tar or arsenic or carbon monoxide, with each dose of nicotine, most people are unintentionally exposing themselves to numerous other chemicals that are known to cause significant long-term health problems. Because of the short duration of action, the increased likelihood of withdrawal symptoms, and the exposure to dangerous chemicals during dosing of the medication, avoiding nicotine use is the best option. If you are a nicotine user, look for ways to stop. There are numerous programs and assistive medications available. Just like with dieting, no one program is perfect for everyone, so you will need to seek out a program that you feel you will be able to live with for the rest of your life. Also, be prepared to try several programs before you find the one that works for you. Persist in your attempts to quit until you're successful, and talk to your doctor about ways she can help.

Caffeine and nicotine are stimulant drugs that are commonly used to increase energy levels; however, there are other medications that are also stimulants that are typically used for other medical conditions. One such medication is **pseudoephedrine**. Pseudoephedrine has a more potent effect on the lining of the nose than caffeine or nicotine. Otherwise, it demonstrates many of the same properties as the other stimulants—most importantly, it improves mental alertness. Pseudoephedrine comes in a variety of different tablet sizes as well as in a liquid form. As with other stimulants, pregnant women and people with heart conditions should avoid taking pseudoephedrine. If you have any questions about any of your particular medical conditions, always discuss the safety of taking any medication with your doctor. The normal dose of pseudoephedrine would be not more than 240mg per day. For example, if you were to use the 12-hour, 120mg tablet, that would be one tablet two times per day. For the smaller, 30mg tablets, that would be 2 tablets every 6 hours. As with other stimulants, the side effects from pseudoephedrine include nervousness, agitation, and increased blood pressure. Pseudoephedrine can cause withdrawal symptoms when taken on a regular basis and then stopped abruptly, and it can affect sleep just like other stimulants. The different forms of pseudoephedrine start to show their effects at different times (typically one to two hours after the initial dose), and the duration of action varies from one form to another (typically lasting anywhere from 4-48 hours). One of the unique issues with regards to pseudoephedrine compared to caffeine and nicotine is that it's more difficult to purchase. Over the years, some people were found to be buying pseudoephedrine and converting it into methamphetmines. Because of this abuse, the FDA now requires that all products containing pseudoephedrine be sold through a pharmacy counter. For now, you do not need a prescription from your doctor to buy pseudoephedrine, but in most states you'll need to present your driver's license to the pharmacist in order to make your purchase, and the pharmacist will only be able to sell you a certain quantity of the medication each day. Despite these limitations, overall, pseudoephedrine provides a relatively convenient way for people to get extra energy, with limited side effects. Again, track your intake diary and your sleep diary to see how each dose of pseudoephedrine is affecting your sleep efficiency, and be sure to discuss any questions or concerns about taking pseudoephedrine or any stimulant with your doctor or pharmacist, ideally before you begin taking the medications and definitely if you experience any unexpected side effects.

Besides the common pharmaceuticals used to increase energy, there is a very wide array of herbal supplements touted to improve energy and alertness as well. I will now review some of these herbs and what information I could find about their effects. The **California poppy** (Eschscholtzia californica) is commonly used for fatigue. I could not find any good information about how or why it's used, but I did find several articles recommending its use for fatigue. I'm always cautious when using any medication that has a limited amount of good information about it readily available, so I'd avoid taking California poppy until more information is available about its effects and its side effects.

Ginkgo biloba is a tree whose leaves and seeds are often dried and ground and used in teas and capsules to help promote blood flow to the brain. This medication appears to have some blood thinning properties, and it may dilate or open up arteries to allow increased blood flow to certain parts of the body as well. The typical dose of ginkgo is 120 to 240mg per dose, typically given 2 or 3 times per day. Overall, the research suggests that there is improved mental alertness in those taking ginkgo. The primary side effect appears to be an increased risk of bleeding, especially in those who are also taking blood thinners. **Ginseng** and **Siberian ginseng** are herbs commonly used to help with low energy levels. The form of ginseng typically used is produced from the root of the ginseng plants (Panax ginseng). This is a different plant than Siberian ginseng (Eleutherococcus senticosus), but the overall effects of the two medications appear to be similar. The typical dose of ginseng is 1-2 grams per day while for Siberian ginseng it is 2-3 grams per day. The research to date suggests beneficial effects in memory and energy level, although these effects are typically mild. The side effects of these products are predominantly related to the stimulant effects of the medications with elevated blood pressure and nervousness predominating. **Mate** (Ilex paraguariensis) is a plant whose leaves and stems contain caffeine. The normal dose of this plant is three grams per day, and it can be taken either as a tea or a capsule. The medicinal effects as well as the side effects are similar to those mentioned above for caffeine. **Spinach** (Spinacia oleracea) is a plant whose leaves are commonly used to reduce fatigue. Spinach contains significant amounts of iron, and, although there appear to be no good scientific studies of its effectiveness to help with fatigue, I would expect it to help with anemia in a person who is not already taking in adequate levels of iron supplementation.

Now that we've finished our review of some of the medications commonly used to increase energy, let's take a look at some medications that are commonly used to help us relax or sleep. When looking at over-the-counter medications that are promoted as sleep aids or suggest that they help us fall asleep, most of these contain antihistamines (anti-allergy medications). Historically, people who suffered with allergy symptoms had few effective treatment options, so they would take antihistamines whenever the symptoms became too severe. Unfortunately, most of the older antihistamines caused significant drowsiness as a side effect, and this drowsiness was severe enough that it limited the frequency and the situations in which people were willing and able to take them. In time, two medical developments occurred in response to the drowsiness noted with the classic antihistamines: some drug companies produced non-sedating antihistamines so people could treat their allergies and still function during the daytime hours, and other drug companies took the older antihistamines and started selling them for another use—as sleep aids. The sedating antihistamine that is most commonly sold as a sleep aid is **diphenhydramine**. Diphenhydramine is the active ingredient in most of the "PM" medications and others that are sold as sleep aids. When trying to decide whether or not to take the older antihistamines to help with sleep, I'd encourage you to consider the fact that diphenhydramine and other sedating antihistamines do, in fact, make people drowsy, but they also tend to adversely influence our brains' normal sleep cycles. Somewhat similar to the effect of alcohol, we might feel drowsy when we take OTC sleep medications, but our brains will experience reduced deep sleep and reduced REM sleep, and we will find that our sleep is less refreshing. As we tracked alcohol in our intake diary, I'd encourage you to do the same tracking when taking OTC sleep medications. Most people will find that their sleep will be more refreshing without these medications and that utilizing some of the other techniques we discussed earlier (e.g. good sleep hygiene, avoiding bedtime stimulation, relaxation before bed) will provide much better long-term results.

Besides the common pharmaceuticals, there are several herbal supplements that are commonly used to help with relaxation and/or sleep. **Valerian root** (valeriana officinalis) is a plant whose roots are ground to make both an oil and a powder. These substances are often used in teas as well as bath oils to help promote relaxation and induce sleep. There is some research that suggests that valerian root can be helpful in promoting sleep, but the overall effect on sleep architecture isn't well studied. **Melatonin** is a hormone that is naturally produced by our brains, and its main role is to regulate our circadian rhythms (although there may be other functions that have not been discovered yet). Melatonin supplements are available in the United States, and while some supplements may contain melatonin taken from animal brains (pigs in particular), most are synthetic versions of the hormone. Several studies have been done on the use of melatonin to treat a variety of different sleep disorders including chronic insomnia and jet lag, but to date, the benefits have been small and there have been several cases of moderate to severe side effects associated with prolonged use. At this point in time, melatonin is considered a nutritional supplement and is not regulated by the FDA; however, due to the relative lack of information about the benefits and risks associated with long-term use, working closely with your doctor on the dosage, frequency, and duration of therapy is the safest way to use melatonin to help with sleep disorders.

Since insomnia is often one of the many symptoms people experience when they are dealing with anxiety or depression, treating these mood disorders often helps improve sleep patterns, and there are several herbal supplements that are commonly used to help these conditions. **St. John's wort** (Hypericum perforatum) is a plant that is used to treat depression and anxiety. It can be taken as a tea or in a capsule. Several studies have been done that have shown it to be effective in treating mild to moderate depression. It is thought to work on the serotonin, norepinephrine, and dopamine levels in the brain. Usual doses can range from 300mg to 4 grams (which is the same as 4000mg) per day. Side effects are generally limited, although it can enhance the side effects typically experienced with other antidepressant medications if it is taken at the same time. **5-hydroxytryptophan (5-HTP)** and **brewer's yeast** (that contains **L-tryptophan** which is converted to 5-HTP in our bodies) are herbal supplements commonly used to treat a variety of different medical conditions from insomnia to depression. Once 5-HTP enters our bloodstreams, it is converted to serotonin in our brains. We discussed serotonin's effects earlier, and serotonin, at certain levels, is known to improve depression and anxiety and can cause drowsiness. Unfortunately, the conversion from 5-HTP to serotonin happens at different rates in different people, so the effects and benefits of using 5-HTP are potentially less predictable compared to other medications used to increase serotonin levels. For this reason, there are probably better options if your goal is to increase the serotonin levels in your brain. However, if you've tried the other medications without success, 5-HTP or brewer's yeast may be reasonable alternatives.

Most of these herbal supplements have been used for centuries and are still being used by many people in the U.S. and abroad. As we discussed earlier, always remember that herbal preparations are typically not regulated or controlled by any government or independent 3rd-party agency. Since herbal supplements are considered food products, there are no standards requiring any level of consistency from capsule to capsule. Each capsule, whether made by the same manufacturer or by different manufacturers, may have a different amount of the stated medication in it. In other words, one capsule could have twice the amount of active ingredient in it compared to another capsule, even in the same bottle. Vitamin and herbal supplement manufacturers are allowed to have tremendous variation from capsule to capsule, and there can even be significantly different forms of a medication from one brand to the next. One manufacturer may get their herbs from China and another may get theirs from Brazil. As with coffee and tea and grapes and other edible plants that are grown around the world, the soil and temperature and rain and agricultural practices in each part of the world can lead to vastly different crops harvested from each point on the globe. Just as some coffees or teas or wines are stronger than others, some herbs grown in certain parts of the world may be stronger than others. The relative strength of an herb is important both in terms of what dose is required to achieve the desired effect and what dose causes unexpected side effects. These side effects are not monitored by the FDA or anyone else in particular, and it's not until a trend towards severe adverse outcomes occurs that the government steps in and removes or restricts the use of a supplement (as was the case with **kava** in 2002 and **mau-huang** in 2004). Until that point, these medications can be sold with few restrictions. Even more concerning is the fact that manufacturers can promote their herbal products as being valid treatments for nearly any disease they decide to put on their labels, whether the supplement actually works for a particular condition or not. Many of the claims on the labels of vitamin and herbal supplements are either based on very limited research or on no research at all. Yet they may contain powerful medications that have potent effects, side effects, and interactions with other medications you might be taking. With that said, before taking any new supplement, I would strongly suggest you discuss its medicinal effects with either your pharmacist or your doctor. Once you feel it's safe to take, look for a reputable manufacturer who guarantees standardized amounts of active ingredients among the capsules in each bottle, as well as from bottle to bottle. Also look for lot numbers and dates of manufacture that can act as safety identification numbers if the manufacturer discovers problems with a certain batch of their medication and needs to withdraw it from the market.

Besides these over-the-counter medications commonly used to increase energy levels, there is a wide variety of prescription medications your doctor may choose to try for you. As with all medications, there is always the potential for side effects, withdrawal, and abuse, so most doctors use these prescription medications with great caution. If you have severe fatigue, have tried everything else we have discussed to this point, and have been evaluated by your doctor without identifying another cause of fatigue, discuss the option of prescription medications to treat your fatigue with your doctor. There are numerous medications your doctor may choose for you. I recommend that you be as aware as possible of the effects and side effects of each medication before starting it. For the most part these days, when a pharmacist fills a prescription, he also attaches an information sheet about the medication. Spend a few minutes with your pharmacist to review the information sheet before taking the medication for the first time. If your pharmacist doesn't routinely give you information, ask him for some or ask your doctor. Drug interactions are also important. You may want to be sure that your doctor or your pharmacist has searched for drug interactions between your current medications and any new prescriptions you receive. You may want to find out if your doctor has a way of checking for drug interactions before writing you a new prescription. Finally, **drug errors** are a common cause of problems for those taking medications. When you receive your prescription, review the name of the medication and what your pharmacist says it is usually used for. If you've been taking the medication for a while, double check to be sure the pills you are receiving look like the pills you've received in the past. If you think you received the wrong medication, don't be shy about reviewing things with your pharmacist. I have had patients receive a new generic tablet (no problem), and I have had patients receive the wrong drug even though the label on the bottle was for the correct drug (big problem). I've seen medication errors happen numerous times. I had a patient receive hydrocortisone (a steroid) when he should have received hydrochlorothiazide (a diuretic). He didn't notice the mistake until he had been taking the wrong medication for two months and noticed his blood pressure was going up instead of down. I had a patient who was prescribed a medication for anxiety. The label on the bottle was correct, but the pills in the bottle were diuretics. Instead of feeling less anxious, the patient was feeling worse because he was urinating constantly and becoming dehydrated. There is no fool-proof method to ensure you get the correct medication, and you are the last person to double check before you finally put it into your body. You have the ability to help reduce medication errors, and I would encourage you to be vigilant in the process.

In this final section of this chapter, I am going to review the effects and side effects of some of the medications doctors prescribe every day. We use numerous prescription medications that either treat fatigue or that can cause fatigue. It would be prohibitive for me to go through all of these (that's why we have 3000 page books as references), but I would like to review some of the general categories of medications we use as well as what we use them for and some of their most common side effects. Again, this list is not meant to be exhaustive, so if you don't see a medication listed here and you have questions about it, please ask your doctor.

The first general category of medications I would like to discuss is preparations that help us to go to sleep. Over the years, we have used many different drugs for this. Included are antihistamines such as Benadryl®, antidepressants such as Elavil® and Desyrel®, medications for anxiety such as Xanax® and Ativan®, and compounds specifically designed for sleep such as Ambien® and Sonata®. At this point in time, there is a fair amount of controversy over which of these medications is the best and the safest. Most of them can cause significant impairment in mental function which, especially in the elderly, can lead to falls and potential injuries. Many can cause sedation that lingers into the following day, causing the person to feel hung over and possibly even making it dangerous for them to drive. Also, many of these are habit-forming, meaning that if used on a consistent basis, your body may get used to them and you may feel even worse when you stop using them. Overall, I recommend you discuss the options with your doctor and/or your pharmacist, but whichever medication you end up using to help you sleep, I would encourage you to be aware of the side effects and try to limit your usage to the minimum amount absolutely necessary.

The next general category of medications we use to treat fatigue-causing illnesses include those for depression. As we've discussed, it's a lower-than-normal level of serotonin in the brain that leads to depression; therefore, antidepressants increase the functional levels of serotonin within our brains. Medications such as Paxil®, Prozac®, Zoloft®, Wellbutrin®, Elavil®, and Celexa® all do this. Each medication can increase the serotonin level to a different extent, and each has the potential to increase the functional effects of other chemicals in the brain as well. The range of side effects seen by people taking these medications is quite varied, but in general we tend to see some side effects more commonly than others. One of the most common is feeling disconnected and having a difficult time focusing attention. This is especially noticeable for the first week or two when starting the medication or when increasing the dosage. We often see increased nervousness, headaches, and stomach upset when starting these medications. Some patients feel increased fatigue with their first few doses while others notice increased energy levels. The most concerning issue for many of my patients is a change in sex drive or difficulty having an orgasm while taking these medications. Some patients gain weight with these medications while other patients lose weight. In rare cases, severe side effects, like increased thoughts of suicide, have occurred. Many of these side effects do go away if a person can manage to get through the first few weeks of taking the medication, but nowadays there is such a wide variety of medications in this category to choose from that we often can find one that treats the depression and leaves the person with very limited, very tolerable side effects.

The final general category I would like to discuss is medications we use to treat blood pressure. Interestingly enough, many of the same medications used to treat hypertension are also used for congestive heart failure. These include preparations that cause the heart to beat more slowly and less forcefully such as atenolol, metoprolol, Norvasc®, and Procardia®. As you might expect, they can make us feel more tired because they are reducing the amount of blood the heart is pumping out with each beat. Besides their effects on the heart, they also have some effect on the blood vessels themselves, causing them to relax and accept more blood with each heartbeat. This has the overall effect of lowering blood pressure. These medications can also cause fluid retention and swelling which are related to the relaxation of the blood vessels. Slowed heart beat and fluid retention both tend to make us feel more sluggish and fatigued.

Other medications such as Univasc®, Lotensin®, and Altace® cause blood vessels to relax and accept more blood with each heartbeat as well. They also inhibit the kidneys from retaining salt and water. Diuretics such as Lasix® and hydrochlorothiazide also cause us to put out excess salt and water into our urine. All of these medications have the potential side effect of causing chemical imbalances, especially in regards to sodium and potassium. They can also have harmful effects on the kidneys themselves, so routine blood tests are required to monitor kidney function while we are taking them. Furthermore, a chronic state of dehydration is one of the goals of these medications, so chronic fatigue can easily follow due to the excessive water loss into the urine.

There are other medications we could discuss if we had time, but I think this list at least gets us started thinking about some of the most commonly-used and some of their side effects. Whether you are on one of these medications or on another not listed here, you will get the best and most complete information about the effects and side effects from either you pharmacist or your doctor. I strongly encourage you to review your medications and become familiar with the potential side effects. This may be the final clue you need in your effort to find the cause of your fatigue.

The only other treatment for fatigue I would like to review in more detail is that used for **obstructive sleep apnea**. As you recall, obstructive sleep apnea is caused by the extra tissues in the back of the throat collapsing over and covering the opening to your lungs. There are several treatments that are important to mention. First of all, obstructive sleep apnea tends to be worse when a person sleeps on his back, so forcing him to sleep on his side or stomach can often improve sleep quality. We can "force" him to sleep on his side by using a pillow behind him when he sleeps, making it more difficult to roll over onto his back at night. We can also use a tennis ball strategically positioned under the sheets so that when the person does roll back, he quickly become uncomfortable and rolls onto his side or stomach again. There are surgical techniques occasionally used to treat sleep apnea. With these procedures, the surgeon removes some tissues from the back of the throat. Unfortunately, to this point, it has only provided limited improvement in frequency and duration of apnea episodes. Continued research and improved procedures may prove more effective in the future. One of the most globally beneficial means for treating obstructive sleep apnea is through weight loss. A relatively moderate degree of weight loss (20-30 pounds) can have a profound effect on the occurrences of apnea. This method of treating obstructive sleep apnea clearly has the fewest side effects and the most benefits for our overall health, but losing 20-30 pounds can often present a tremendous challenge. Finally, and most importantly, the most effective treatment for obstructive sleep apnea is the **continuous positive airway pressure machine (CPAP machine)**. A CPAP machine uses a face mask that covers either just the nose or both the nose and the mouth. Into this face mask, air is blown with a certain amount of pressure. The pressure pushes the tissues in the back of the throat out of the way so air can flow freely into the lungs. CPAP isn't the easiest treatment to get used to. In fact, I frequently have patients complain about how uncomfortable their face masks are; however, there is a wide variety of shapes and sizes of face masks. Usually almost all of the discomfort can be alleviated by finding the proper face mask. Once the face mask fits and the CPAP machine is allowed to work, the results can be spectacular, and many patients notice they haven't slept that well and they haven't felt that energetic in years.

Other Treatment Options

Chapter 10: Final Thoughts

If you feel fine, keep doing whatever you're doing. When I see a 90-year-old smoker in my office who hasn't seen a doctor in 20 years and is only there because he developed a rash that he can't get rid of, I can't argue with his lifestyle at all. Whatever he's doing is working for him. But if you are not feeling up to doing the things you want to be doing, consider making some of the changes discussed in this book.

Fatigue is clearly a confounding issue. Incredible numbers of people suffer from it on a routine basis, and the numbers are only increasing as more and more of us are working harder and are being given more responsibilities in our daily lives. For many, the only means of dealing with their fatigue is to try to live around it. They are constantly adjusting their lives so they can fit their fatigue into their increasingly-busy schedules, but somehow, fatigue always seems to win out, and they may miss many of the enjoyable parts of life due to a lack of energy. Fortunately, fatigue doesn't have to control us. We can figure out the causes of our fatigue in most cases, and once we know why we are fatigued, correcting the problem becomes possible. The steps we must take in order to correct our energy deficit may sound challenging. The truth is that they are really quite manageable. If we can convince ourselves that we are tired of being tired and that we want to have more energy to do the things we want to do, we can find the focus necessary to make the strides towards feeling better. Once you understand what you have to do to correct your fatigue, you will have to confront many of your old habits and determine how valuable they are. Is it worthwhile spending several hours each day watching television? How important are cigarettes? How difficult would it be to incorporate exercise into your daily schedule? Can you find a way to lose weight? Should you visit your doctor to discuss your problems? These are questions only you can answer, and when seeking the answers, you will have to compare the difficulties in taking these steps to what you could accomplish if you had as much energy as you wanted.

As you confront your fatigue and take on the challenge of treating it, I wish you good luck and good health.

James C. Gariti, M.D.

Glossary of Terms

% Daily Value—a number printed on food and vitamin supplement labels that is designed to tell us what percentage of the total recommended amount of each nutrient is contained in one serving of the food or vitamin you are taking

5-hydroxytryptophan (5-HTP)—an herb used to treat anxiety and depression

Acquired immunodeficiency syndrome (AIDS)—an infection with the human immunodeficiency virus (HIV) which is characterized by decreased function of the immune system

Actigraph—a machine used to measure body movement

Adrenal glands—small clusters of cells that sit on top of the kidneys and produce a variety of different hormones

Adrenaline (AKA epinephrine)—a stimulant our bodies produce in response to stress

Aerobic exercise—exercise that increases a person's heart rate and causes the person to breathe more rapidly and more deeply than normal

Allergens—chemicals that cause a person's immune system to overreact, leading to the release of the chemicals of inflammation

Allergist and immunologist—a doctor who specialize in evaluating and treating allergic conditions

Alveous (plural is alveoli)—a small air space within the lung tissue

Anemia—a situation in which the blood does not have enough of the oxygen-carrying component, hemoglobin

Anesthesiologist—a doctor who specializes in relieving pain

Angina—a situation in which not enough oxygen and nutrients are getting to the heart muscle leading to pain in the heart muscle without actually injuring the heart muscle

Angioplasty—a procedure in which a very small, deflated balloon is attached to the end of a wire, the balloon is placed in the

179

center of a stenotic segment of coronary artery (something like putting a piece of thread through the eye of a needle), the balloon is then blown up, and as the balloon expands, it stretches and eventually breaks the stenosis

Antibiotic resistance—a situation in which bacteria learn how to not be killed by certain antibiotics

Antibody—one of the chemicals released by the body's immune system that is specifically designed to attack a particular antigen

Antigen—a chemical that enters the body and stimulates an immune response

Antinuclear antibody (ANA)—a blood test used to look for signs of autoimmune diseases

Antiretroviral medications—antibiotic-like medicines that fight against certain viruses

Aplastic anemia—the form of anemia caused by the bone marrow not producing enough red blood cells

Arteries—the blood vessels that carry blood away from the heart

Ascites—fluid accumulation in the belly as a result of liver failure

Asthma—a medical condition in which chronic irritation of the lungs leads to chronic inflammation, mucous production, and thickening of the air tubes

Attention deficit hyperactivity disorder (ADHD)—a medical condition in which a person's brain is too active and the brain bounces from one idea to the next without the person being able to always control when and where the thoughts bounce

Autoimmune disease—a disease in which the body mistakenly views itself as an enemy leading the immune system to attack and destroy itself

Basophil—a sub type of white blood cell that is involved in allergic responses

Benign prostatic hypertrophy (BPH)—a medical condition in which the prostate enlarges and it squeezes the bladder neck and blocks the urine from coming out of the bladder

Bile—a green liquid produced by the liver that not only excretes waste into the intestines but also helps break down fat that is passing through the intestines

Bilirubin—a chemical that is put out in bile

Bio-identical hormones—hormones that are commercially produced and are designed to "look" just like the hormones that are produced by a woman's ovaries

Bladder neck—the bottom of the bladder

Blood-brain barrier (BBB)—a filter surrounding the brain that only lets certain chemicals that are floating around in the blood enter the brain

Blood pressure—the amount of pressure in our blood vessels, measured before and after our heart squeezes blood into them

Blood vessels—tubes that hold the blood within the body

Body mass index (BMI)—a ratio of weight (in kilograms) divided by height (in meters)^2

Bone marrow—cells in the middle of our bones that have starter cells that can produce numerous new blood cells

Bone mineral density (BMD)—a measurement of bone strength

Borrelia burgdorferi—the bacteria that cause Lyme disease

Botulinum toxin—an "all-natural" product that is one of the most potent nerve toxins ever discovered

Brewer's yeast—an herb used to treat anxiety and depression

C-reactive protein (CRP)—a blood test used to measure inflammation in the body

Caffeine—a stimulant chemical present in coffee, tea, soda, and other foods

Calcitonin—a hormone the body releases when it senses that the blood calcium levels are getting too high which stimulates the extra calcium to enter the bones

Calcium—an electrolyte that is used for muscle and nerve function and that is stored in the bones

California poppy—an herb used to treat fatigue

Cancer—the abnormal growth of cells in the body that eventually leads to uncontrolled growth and spread of these abnormal cells beyond the location they should normally stay

Carbon dioxide—a normal waste product our bodies produce as they use glucose for energy

Carbon monoxide—a waste product generated when something like natural gas or wood is burned

Carbon monoxide poisoning—a medical condition caused by exposure to excessive levels of carbon monoxide that can lead to symptoms such as nausea, headache, sleepiness

Cardiologist—a doctor who specializes in diagnosing and treating diseases of the heart

Cardiothoracic surgeon—a doctor who specializes in doing surgery on the heart

Cardiovascular exercise—exercise that elevates a person's heart rate and gets the person to the point that she needs to breathe more deeply and more rapidly than normal in order to keep doing the exercise

Cell—the building blocks of the body. They are analogous to the individual bricks that are the building blocks of a house.

Central sleep apnea—a condition in which our brain does not sense the need to take a breath while asleep, so despite falling oxygen levels, our brain does not tell us to take a breath

Chemotactic factors—an immune mediator

Chiropractors—a doctor who specializes in the movement of the body

Chronic bronchitis—see chronic obstructive pulmonary disease

Chronic fatigue syndrome—a disease that is characterized by long-term fatigue which interferes with life and is not caused by another medical condition. The cause of chronic fatigue syndrome is unknown

Chronic obstructive pulmonary disease (COPD)—a disease in which lung tissue is slowly eaten away (commonly caused by cigarette smoking)

Circadian rhythm—our internal clock that controls our body's functions based on the night/day cycle

Cirrhosis—a medication condition in which enough scar tissue forms within the liver that a person develops liver failure

Complete blood count (CBC)—a blood test that measures the various cells in our blood

Compliment—an immune mediator

Compounding pharmacy—a pharmacy that essentially makes its own medications

Comprehensive metabolic panel (CMP)—a blood test used to measure numerous chemicals in the blood

Concentration—the ability to focus one's mind in order to complete a task

Congestive heart failure (CHF)—a disease in which the heart cannot pump enough blood forward through the body, so the blood backs up

Continuous positive airway pressure machine (CPAP machine)—a machine that pushes the tissues in the back of the throat out of the way by forcing air into the nose and mouth

Contraction—the squeezing action of the heart muscle

Coronary arteries—the arteries that carry fresh blood into the heart muscle itself

Cortisol—a type of glucocorticoid

Crohn's disease—an autoimmune disease in which the immune system attacks the intestines

Cytokines—an immune mediator

Dehydration—a situation in which the body does not contain as much water as it should

Delusion—having strong beliefs that something is true even when given facts proving that it is not true

Deoxyribonucleic acid (DNA)—a blueprint our cells use to guide the construction of each cell in our bodies

Depressant—a chemical that slows down brain function

Diabetes mellitus (or just "diabetes")—a medical condition in which the amount of glucose floating around in the blood is too high

Dialysis—a method of removing waste products from the blood of a person who has kidney failure. This method involves passing a person's blood through a machine that filters out all the waste products.

Diastole—the portion of the heart beat when the heart muscle is relaxing

Diastolic blood pressure—bottom number recorded in a blood pressure reading that represents is the lowest amount of pressure that remains in the arteries when the heart is relaxing during diastole

Diastolic dysfunction—the type of congestive heart failure that results when the heart muscle cannot relax enough to allow a normal amount of blood to enter it

Dietician—a professional who can evaluate what a person is eating and make suggestion about ways of improving the nutritional value of the food they eat

Dilute—to water down

Diphenhydramine—an older allergy medication that causes drowsiness and is, therefore, used in many sleep aids

Diuretic—any medication that causes us to put out excess water into our urine

Dopamine—a chemical present in the synapses of the brain that allows the passage of information from one part of the brain to another.

Echinacea—an herbal supplement commonly used to treat colds

Echocardiogram (or "echo")—an ultrasound of the heart used to evaluate the structure and function of the heart

Eczema—an allergic reaction leading to inflammation of the skin

Electrocardiogram (or "ECG" or "EKG")—the printout that shows the pattern of movement of electricity through the heart muscle

Electrocardiograph—a machine designed to measure the movement of electricity through the heart muscle

Electrolytes—various salts like sodium, potassium, calcium, magnesium, and chloride

Emphysema—see chronic obstructive pulmonary disease

Endocrinologist—a doctor who specializes in diagnosing and treating abnormalities of the body's hormonal system

Endorphins—chemicals our bodies produce that make us relax and feel happy

Enzymes—proteins within the body that perform various jobs

Eosinophil—a sub type of white blood cell that is involved in allergic responses as well as in fighting fungal and parasitic infections

Epinephrine—a chemical present in the synapses of the brain that allows the passage of information from one part of the brain to another. This chemical is also present in the blood and is released in response to stress and is part of the fight or flight response.

Epstein-Barr virus (or EBV)—the virus that causes mononucleosis

Erythropoietin—the hormone produced by the kidney that stimulates red blood cell production

Erythrocyte sedimentation rate (ESR)—a blood test used to measure levels of inflammation

Exercise stress test—a test designed to evaluate blood flow to the heart muscle which is typically performed by having a person walk on a treadmill while monitoring heart activity

Exhale—the portion of the breathing cycle during which we breathe out

Fatigue—weariness or exhaustion from labor, exertion, or stress

Fibromyalgia—a disease characterized by diffuse body aches and tenderness which interfere with normal life functions. The cause of fibromyalgia is unknown.

Fight or flight response—when we are faced with a life-threatening situation, our brains and our bodies are hardwired to either fight against the threat or run away from the threat

Folate (or folic acid)—a nutrient used by our bodies to build and maintain DNA

Fructose—the form of sugar found in fruits

Ginkgo biloba—an herb used to increased blood flow to the brain

Ginseng—an herb used to treat fatigue

Glucagon—a hormone produced by the pancreas during times of low blood glucose that stimulates fat cells to be converted to glucose as well as liver cells to release more glucose

Glucocorticoids—a type of hormone produced by the body during periods of stress which reduce levels of inflammation in the body

Glucometer—a machine that measures the amount of glucose in the blood

Glucose—the form of sugar our bodies can use for energy

Glycogen—a chemical, which is like a stack of glucose molecules all clumped together, used by the liver to store excess energy

Granuloma—a ball of scar tissue that forms around bacteria, typically in the lungs, which prevents the immune system and antibiotics from reaching and attacking the bacteria

Hallucination—seeing or hearing things that aren't really there

Heart attack—see myocardial infarction

Hematologist/oncologist—a doctor who specializes in diagnosing and treating medical problems of the blood (hematology) as well as diagnosing and treating cancers (oncology)

Hematology—the study of medicine related to problems of the blood

Hematopoiesis—the process of producing more RBCs along with the other cells in the blood

Hemoglobin—the chemical inside the red blood cell that carries oxygen

Hemolytic anemia—anemia that results from the premature destruction of RBCs

Hepatitis—an inflammation of the liver caused by chemicals or infection

Home oxygen monitor—a test that can be performed in a person's home that monitors the person's oxygen levels while they sleep

Hormone—a chemical released by one part of our body that sends a signal to the rest of the body stimulating the other part of the body to perform a certain function

Hormone replacement therapy (HRT)—hormones given to a person with the intention of replacing the hormones the body is no longer producing. The hormones commonly given in replacement therapy include estrogen, progesterone, and testosterone.

Human immunodeficiency virus (HIV)—a virus that attacks the body's immune system, making the immune system less effective

Hypertension—a situation in which the amount of pressure in the blood vessels is higher than it should be

Hypoglycemia—a state of low blood glucose levels

Hyponatremia—a state of low levels of sodium in the blood

Hypotension—a situation in which the amount of pressure in the blood vessels is lower than it should be

Hyperthyroidism—a medical condition in which the level of thyroid hormone is higher than normal

Hypothyroidism—a medical condition in which the level of thyroid hormone is lower than normal

Immunoglobulin—an immune mediator

Immunosuppressants—medications designed to reduce our bodies' immune responses

Infectious disease specialist—a doctor who specializes in detecting and treating many illnesses caused by infections

Inflammation—the body's response to irritation

Inflammatory mediators—the chemicals that are released as part of the body's response to irritation

Insomnia—the inability to fall asleep

Insulin—the hormone our bodies produce that helps glucose pass into our cells so that our cells can use the glucose as an energy source

Insulin dependent diabetes mellitus (IDDM)—see type I diabetes mellitus

Intake diary—a journal used to keep track of everything taken into our bodies, including, food, drink, and medications

Iron—a chemical that is involved in hematopoiesis

Iron toxicity—a dangerous situation in which a person eats too much iron causing potential injury to the person's body

Jaundice—the result of bilirubin levels rising that leads to the whites of the eyes and the skin developing a yellow color

Jet lag—a shift in the timing of sleep due to travel that results in our bodies feeling like they are in one time zone while our brains feel like they are in another

Kava kava—an "all-natural" anxiety relieving herb that has been linked to increased risk of liver injury and even liver failure

Kidney—the body part that creates urine as it filters the blood and removes waste products from the blood

L-tryptophan—an herb used to treat anxiety and depression

Leukemia—a cancer of the white blood cells

Leukotrienes—an immune mediator

Liver—an organ in the body that filters the blood, removing and metabolizing many waste products from the blood

Liver failure—a medical condition in which the liver is no longer able to perform its normal level of blood filtration and protein production

Lyme disease—a constellation of symptoms including rash, arthritis, and fatigue caused by the Borrelia burgdorferi bacteria

Lymph—the fluid that leaks out of the blood vessels and typically carries a variety of different chemicals including immune cells

Lymph nodes—clusters of immune cells located in all parts of the body—most prominently in the groin, in the armpits, and in the neck—that filter the blood and the lymph

Lymphocyte—a sub type of white blood cell that is primarily responsible for fighting off viral infections

Mania (adjective manic)—a medical condition in which a person has an uncontrollable amount of energy that can keep him from sleeping at night and can cause him to make decisions and take actions he wouldn't normally do

Massage therapist—a person who performs massage which can help reduce muscle tension and help improve relaxation

Mate—a caffeine-containing herb used to treat fatigue

Mau-huang—an "all-natural" stimulating herb that has been linked to increased risk of heart injury

Melatonin—a hormone produced in our brains that promotes sleep and regulates circadian rhythms

Metabolize—to break down or "digest" chemicals in the blood

Monocyte—a sub type of white blood cell that is a supportive cell which helps with the identification of unwanted items into the body and digestion of these unwanted items

Mononucleosis—a disease characterized by severe fatigue and enlarged lymph nodes caused by the Epstein-Barr virus

Multivitamin—a tablet that contains a variety of different vitamins and minerals which is used to supplement a person's daily nutrition

Murmur—a sound made by the heart that is heard when listening to the sounds of the heart

Muscle weakness—not physically being able to perform routine tasks

Mycobacterium tuberculosis—the bacteria that cause tuberculosis infections

Myocardial infarction (MI)—a medical condition in which a segment of the heart muscle does not receive enough blood leading to death of the muscle cells in that segment of the heart

Neurologist—a doctor who specializes in detecting and treating disorders of the nerves and brain

Neutrophil—a sub type of white blood cell that is primarily responsible for fighting off bacterial infections

Nicotine—a stimulant chemical present in tobacco products

Nightmares—particularly bad dreams that adversely affect a person's sleep

Non-insulin dependent diabetes mellitus (NIDDM)—see type II diabetes mellitus

Norepinephrine—a chemical present in the synapses of the brain that allows the passage of information from one part of the brain to another. This chemical is also present in the blood and is released in response to stress and is part of the fight or flight response.

Nucleus (pleural is nuclei)—the part of a cell that controls the function of the cell

Obesity—body mass index greater than 30

Obstructive sleep apnea (OSA)—a disease in which the tissues in the back of a person's throat collapse when they sleep and block the flow of air into the lungs

Oncology—the study of medicine related to cancer

Opium—an "all-natural" hallucinogen and pain medication with unparalleled addictive potential

Orthostatic hypotension—a situation in which the blood pressure is relatively normal while lying or sitting and in which it drops when a person stands up, typically making the person feel dizzy or lightheaded as soon as she goes from sitting or lying to standing

Osteopenia—a situation in which the amount of calcium in the bones is lower than normal but not quite as low as seen with osteoporosis

Osteoporosis—a decrease in the amounts of calcium in the bones that leads to weakening of the bones which makes them fragile and susceptible to breaking

Output diary—a journal used to track how a person spends their time each day

Overactive bladder—a situation in which the bladder muscles have a hard time relaxing, and as soon as the muscles of the bladder start to stretch, they can spasm

Oxygen—a chemical found in air that our bodies use for energy

Pancreas—the organ in the body that senses glucose levels in the blood and releases insulin and glucagon which help the body use glucose correctly

Parathyroid glands—a collection of four small glands located behind the thyroid gland in the front of the neck that release parathyroid hormone

Parathyroid hormone—a hormone the body releases when it senses that the blood calcium levels are getting too low which stimulates calcium to be released from the bones into the blood

Peek flow testing—a breathing test performed at home used to monitor the status and progression of asthma

Personal trainer—a professional who evaluates a person's needs and develops a specific exercise program to meet those needs

Phlebologist—a medical doctor who specializes in the diagnosis and treatments of problems of the venous system

Physiatrist—a doctor who specializes in restoring people back to normal functional levels after incapacitating events

Physical medicine and rehabilitation doctor (PM&R)—same as physiatrist

Physical therapist—a professional who looks at the way we use our bodies to accomplish our daily tasks

Placebo—a simulated treatment for a medical condition. The treatment has no true effect on the medical condition, but it's designed to make the person think she is receiving an effective treatment. The person may experience a perceived or real improvement in the symptoms. Placebos are commonly used in research studies in order to test which effects and side effects are being caused by a medication and which are being caused by a person's mind.

Platelet—the cell in our blood that causes blood clots and scabs to form

Post-nasal drip—a chronic state of mucous dripping down the back of our throats, often caused by chronic, uncontrolled allergies

Prostaglandins—an immune mediator

Prostate—a gland that wraps around the bottom of the bladder in men

Pseudoephedrine—a stimulant medication that is predominantly used to reduce nasal congestion

Psychiatrist—a doctor who specializes in detecting and treating the chemical abnormalities in the brain that cause changes in thinking or reacting to situations

Psychologist—a professional who is very good at looking at how a person deals with various life situations as well as looking at what types of abnormal life situations a person faces on a daily basis

Pulmonary function testing (PFT)—a breathing test performed in a doctor's office used to monitor lung function

Pulmonologist—a doctor who specializes in diseases of the lungs

Purified protein derivative (PPD)—a screening test for tuberculosis that involves a needle prick on the arm

Rapid Eye Movement (REM) sleep—a phase of sleep during which our minds are very active but our bodies are at rest

Red blood cells (RBC)—the cells in the blood that contain hemoglobin and carry oxygen

Restless leg syndrome (RLS)—a disease characterized by any of a number of sensations including burning, itching, tingling, crawling, or tightening in the legs or arms that make the person feel as if they have to move in order to relieve the symptoms

Rheumatoid arthritis—an autoimmune disease characterized by attack on the joints

Rheumatologist—a doctor who specializes in diagnosing and treating diseases involving inflammation

Rhinitis—inflammation of the nose most often caused by an allergic response

Selective serotonin reuptake inhibitors (SSRIs)—medications that make the serotonin that is in the synapses of the brain stay in those synapses longer than normal

Serotonin—the chemical in the brain that is responsible for passing information from the factual portion to the emotional portion of the brain

Serum—the watery part of blood that makes up 2/3 of the volume of blood

Shift work sleep disorder—when people experience insomnia and fatigue associated with working the night shift

Siberian ginseng—an herb used to treat fatigue

Sleep cycle—sequence of sleep stages that progress from Stage 1 to REM and back again

Sleep deprivation—a pattern of routinely not receiving enough sleep

Sleep diary—a journal of a person's pattern of sleep

Sleep efficiency—a comparison between how rested a person feels to how much time she spent in bed

Sleep hygiene—a practice of only sleeping when and where a person is supposed to

Sleep latency—the amount of time between the time when a person goes to bed and the time the person actually falls asleep

Sleep stages—identifiable patterns of electrical activity within people's brains while they sleep

Sleep study—a test performed in a sleep lab where several components of sleep are monitored while the person sleeps

Social isolation—being separated from interactions with others due to a physical or mental barrier

Spinach—an iron-containing plant used to treat fatigue

Spleen—an organ in our bodies that filters out old, worn-out blood cells

St. John's wort—an herb used to treat anxiety and depression

Stenosis—a situation in which a tube (in particular an artery, a vein, or a heart valve) is a smaller size than or does not open to a normal diameter

Stimulants—chemicals that cause the brain to be more awake

Stress response—in response to a stressful situation, the body releases a variety of chemicals in an attempt to help the body deal with the stressful situation

Stress urinary incontinence—a medical condition in which the bladder empties too easily with minimally-increased pressure in the abdomen

Sucrose—the form of sugar found in table sugar

Synapse—the connection between two nerves or between a nerve and another body part

Systemic lupus erythematosus (SLE)—an autoimmune disease characterized by the body attacking a certain part of each cell of the body

Systole—the part of the heart beat when the heart muscle squeezes the blood out of the heart

Systolic blood pressure—top number recorded in a blood pressure reading that represents the maximum amount of pressure the heart creates in the arteries during systole

Systolic dysfunction—the type of congestive heart failure that results when the heart muscle cannot squeeze enough blood out of it

Tension headache—a headache caused by muscle spasms in the muscles of the head and neck

Thrombocytopenia—having a low level of platelets

Thrombocytosis—having a high level of platelets

Thyroid gland—a small gland located in the front of the neck that releases several hormones that perform various functions within the body

Thyroid hormone—a hormone our bodies produce that enters cells and causes them to use more glucose and oxygen as well as makes them more sensitive to adrenaline

Thyroid stimulating hormone (TSH)—a hormone released by the brain that stimulates the release of thyroid hormone

Travel medicine clinic—a medical office that specializes in diseases associated with travel to foreign countries

Travel medicine doctor—a doctor who specializes in diseases associated with travel to foreign countries

Tuberculosis—an infection, commonly of the lung, cause by the Mycobacterium tuberculosis bacteria

Type I diabetes mellitus—previously known as insulin-dependent diabetes mellitus, this is a state of high glucose levels in the blood due to the body not producing adequate levels of insulin

Type II diabetes mellitus—previously known as non-insulin-dependent diabetes mellitus, this is a state of high glucose levels in the blood due to the body's cells not responding to insulin normally

Universal precautions—a practice of treating everyone and their body fluids as if they might have an infection in an effort to prevent the spread of infections

Urge urinary incontinence—a medical condition in which a spasm within the urinary bladder is powerful enough that some urine may leak out of the bladder

Urinary (or bladder) sphincter—the valve that closes the bladder

Urologist—a medical doctor who specializes in diagnosing and treating diseases of the bladder and kidneys

Valerian root—an herb used to promote relaxation

Valvular incompetence or valvular regurgitation—a situation in which the heart valves don't close all the way

Valvuloplasty—a medical procedure in which we stretch a heart valve open

Veins—the blood vessels that carry blood back into the heart

Viral myocarditis—an infection of the heart muscle with a virus

Vitamin B12—a vitamin that is involved in hematopoiesis

Vitamin D—a chemical that is present in some of the foods we eat and is also produced by our skin when our skin is exposed to sunlight which stimulates the intestines to absorb calcium

Water intoxication—a medical condition caused by drinking a very large amount of water (something along the lines of two gallons) in a very short amount of time (something like one hour) that leads to dilution of the electrolytes in the blood which can be life threatening

White blood cell (WBC)—the type of cell in our blood that is part of our immune system

Window period—a period of time during which the HIV virus is growing and taking hold of the immune system but during which we cannot detect it with our tests

Glossary

Index

Index

Carbon dioxide, 20, 21, 34, 35, 56, 58, 69, 136, 182

Carbon monoxide, 20, 57, 137, 164, 182

Carbon monoxide poisoning, 57, 182

Cardiologist, 37, 43, 44, 45, 139, 182

Cardiothoracic surgeon, 43, 44, 182

Cardiovascular exercise, 73, 182

Cell, 34, 36, 45, 48, 49, 56, 60, 61, 62, 65, 66, 68, 70, 71, 75, 76, 81, 82, 86, 88, 132, 133, 136, 137, 159, 179, 181, 182, 183, 185, 186, 187, 188, 189, 191, 192, 193, 194, 195

Central sleep apnea, 129, 182

Chemotactic factors, 82, 182

Chiropractors, 32, 140, 182

Chronic bronchitis—see chronic obstructive pulmonary disease (COPD)

Chronic fatigue syndrome, 98, 99, 139, 182

Chronic obstructive pulmonary disease (COPD), 21, 22, 130, 139, 182, 184

Circadian rhythm, 7, 10, 12, 168, 182, 188

Cirrhosis, 70, 86, 182

Complete blood count (CBC), 132, 133, 134, 183

Compliment, 82, 183

Compounding pharmacy, 26, 183

Comprehensive metabolic panel (CMP), 136, 183

Concentration, 3, 4, 75, 79, 84, 98, 183

Congestive heart failure (CHF), 21, 35, 36, 38, 40, 42, 44, 97, 130, 139, 173, 183, 184, 194

Continuous positive airway pressure machine (CPAP machine), 129, 175, 183

Contraction, 24, 37, 43, 45, 76, 183

Coronary arteries, 44, 180, 183

Cortisol, 83, 183

C-reactive protein (CRP), 134, 136, 181

Cytokines, 82, 183

D

Dehydration, 30, 41, 47, 51, 52, 62, 111, 116, 117, 134, 136, 153, 162, 174, 183

Delusion, 83, 183

Deoxyribonucleic acid (DNA), 159, 183, 185

Depressant, 15, 183

Diabetes mellitus (or just, 44, 47, 52, 61, 62, 63, 64, 65, 71, 72, 73, 74, 75, 76, 138, 140, 150, 151, 183, 187, 189, 194

Dialysis, 71, 183

Diastole, 36, 39, 184

Diastolic blood pressure, 39, 184

Diastolic dysfunction, 36, 38, 39, 184

Dietician, 120, 140, 152, 157, 184

Dilute, 52, 184

Diphenhydramine, 167, 184

Diuretic, 37, 39, 51, 116, 162, 171, 174, 184

Dopamine, 79, 168, 184

E

Echinacea, 94, 184

Echocardiogram (or, 43, 44, 184

Eczema, 84, 184

Electrocardiogram (or, 45, 184

Electrocardiograph, 45, 184

Electrolytes, 31, 37, 47, 52, 75, 76, 78, 181, 184, 195

Emphysema—see chronic obstructive pulmonary disease (COPD)

Endocrinologist, 140, 184

Endorphins, 18, 184

Enzymes, 60, 184

Eosinophil, 132, 185

Epstein-Barr virus (or EBV), 88, 137, 185, 189

Erythrocyte sedimentation rate (ESR), 134, 136, 185

Erythropoietin, 48, 185

Exercise stress test, 45, 185

Exhale, 50, 69, 185

F

Fatigue, i, ii, 1, 3, 4, 5, 7, 8, 9, 10, 11, 12, 13, 14, 15, 20, 21, 22, 23, 32, 33, 35, 36, 41, 44, 47, 53, 55, 56, 57, 61, 62, 63, 64, 66, 68, 69, 70, 71, 75, 77, 80, 82, 83, 84, 88, 89, 90, 91, 93, 95, 97, 98, 99, 100, 101, 103, 106, 111, 112, 113, 115, 116, 117, 121, 123, 124, 126, 127, 128, 129, 131, 132, 134, 136, 137, 138, 140, 141, 145, 149, 150, 161, 165, 170, 172, 174, 177, 178, 181, 182, 185, 188, 189, 192, 193
Fibromyalgia, 99, 139, 185
Fight or flight response, 17, 185, 189
Folate (or folic acid), 137, 159, 185
Fructose, 64, 149, 185

G

Ginkgo biloba, 28, 166, 185
Ginseng, 28, 166, 185
Glucagon, 65, 185, 190
Glucocorticoids, 83, 84, 183, 186
Glucometer, 64, 66, 186
Glucose, 60, 61, 62, 63, 64, 65, 66, 68, 69, 72, 83, 136, 137, 149, 182, 183, 185, 186, 187, 190, 194
Glycogen, 63, 65, 186
Granuloma, 91, 186

H

Hallucination, 83, 186
Heart attack—see myocardial infarction (MI)
Hematologist/oncologist, 49, 50, 186
Hematology, 49, 186
Hematopoiesis, 49, 157, 186, 187, 195
Hemoglobin, 48, 49, 57, 133, 179, 186, 192
Hemolytic anemia, 50, 186
Hepatitis, 70, 84, 87, 91, 137, 186
Home oxygen monitor, 130, 131, 186

Hormone, 8, 17, 25, 27, 48, 60, 65, 66, 67, 68, 78, 83, 124, 131, 159, 168, 179, 181, 185, 186, 187, 188, 190, 194
Hormone replacement therapy (HRT), 25, 27, 186
Human immunodeficiency virus (HIV), 91, 137, 179, 187, 195
Hypertension, 38, 39, 44, 52, 72, 73, 74, 76, 139, 173, 187
Hyperthyroidism, 68, 187
Hypoglycemia, 63, 64, 65, 187
Hyponatremia, 52, 187
Hypotension, 41, 42, 139, 187
Hypothyroidism, 68, 132, 187

I

Immunoglobulin, 82, 187
Immunosuppressants, 93, 187
Infectious disease specialist, 140, 187
Inflammation, 58, 81, 82, 83, 84, 92, 117, 134, 139, 179, 180, 181, 184, 185, 186, 187, 192
Inflammatory mediators, 58, 67, 81, 82, 84, 92, 124, 187
Insomnia, 11, 13, 14, 19, 161, 168, 187, 192
Insulin, 60, 61, 64, 66, 67, 187, 190, 194
Insulin dependent diabetes mellitus (IDDM)—see type I diabetes mellitus
Intake diary, 115, 116, 117, 118, 120, 121, 122, 128, 138, 162, 165, 167, 187
Iron, 48, 50, 117, 137, 157, 166, 187, 193
Iron toxicity, 158, 187

J

Jaundice, 69, 70, 86, 187
Jet lag, 12, 168, 188

Index

Index

www.ingramcontent.com/pod-product-compliance
Lightning Source LLC
Chambersburg PA
CBHW070643290526
45790CB00001B/175